HEATHER'S HEDGEHOG HOSTEL

Heather's Hedgehog Hostel
ISBN: 9798853373716

Photos courtesy of Heather's Hedgehog Hostel

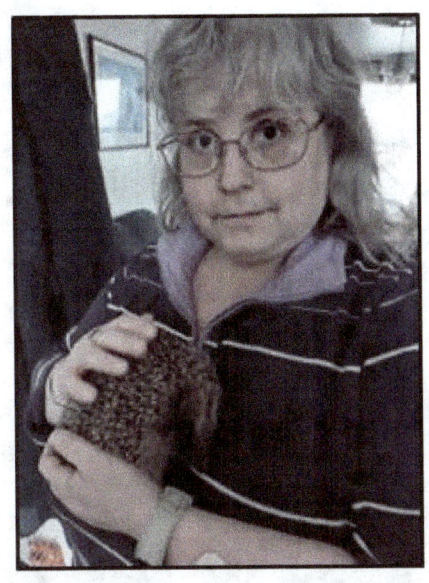

In a quiet little town called Chatteris, you'll find Heather's Hedgehog Hostel

It's not an obvious hostel and you'd probably miss it if you didn't know it was in Heather's house.

Hedgehogs go there when they aren't feeling so prickly, and sometimes she has so many little creatures to look after, she has no time to do anything other than go to her teaching job, eat and sleep.

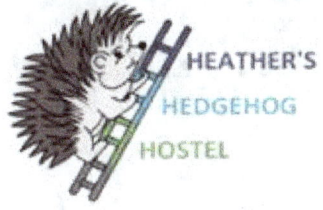

HEATHER'S
HEDGEHOG
HOSTEL

Heather rescues and rehabilitates wild hedgehogs after they've been hurt in some way.

She cleans them up, gives them a place to rest, food, medication and antibiotics.

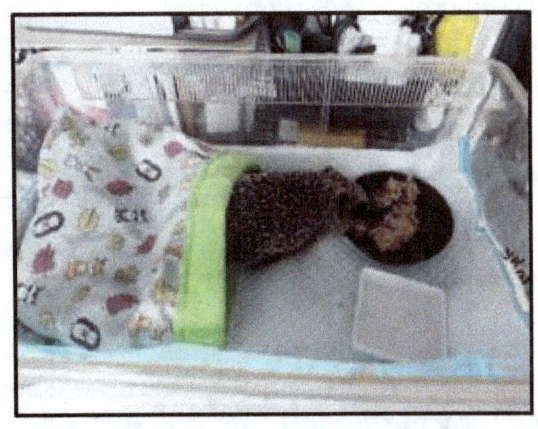

Our native hedgehogs live in the wild and sometimes they get bitten by dogs and foxes, or cut with lawn mowers and grass strimmers.

Occasionally, they even get burned in bonfires, shot, or kicked by cruel people who should know better.

One huge hedgehog came in to the hostel because some cruel boys were using him as a football.

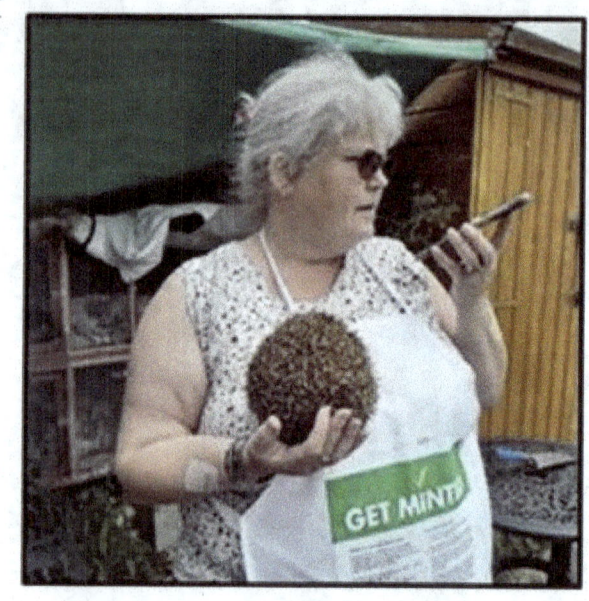

Heather named him Gary.

Then, there are the hedgehogs which suffer from fly strikes, ringworm, or get dehydrated when they can't find anything to drink.

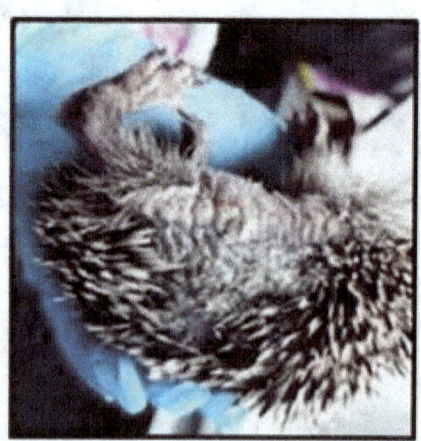

Whatever the reason, Heather is always on hand to give advice and help get the little mammals back on their feet again.

Sometimes, Heather gets babies in. They're really cute, but need a lot of attention.

After the babies have been born in the wild, the new hedgehog mother leaves them to go off and collect food.

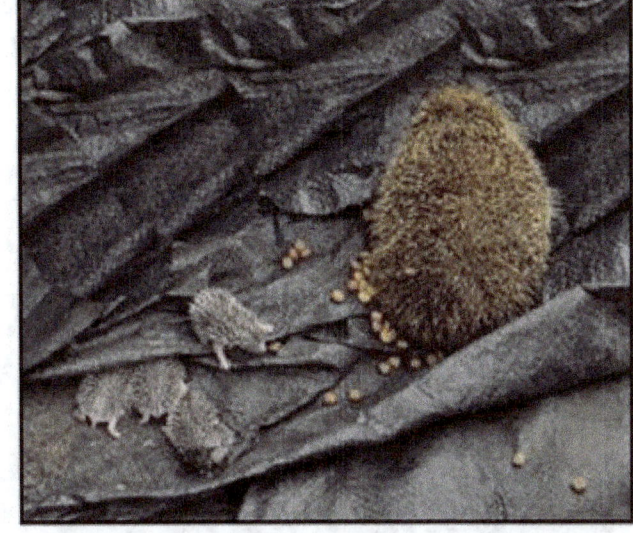

She usually gives birth to four or five babies at a time and her foraging can take up to two hours, so if you find a baby hedgehog nest don't disturb it.

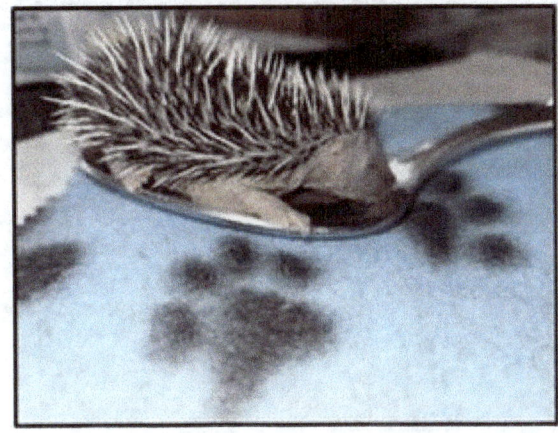

Baby hedgehogs are called hoglets, and have about 100 spines when they're first born.

These are covered with loose skin though, so at first, they look like grey bath brushes.

They're very tiny, and some Heather gets in can even fit on a teaspoon.

The white spikes soon poke through and as the hoglets get bigger, they get more prickles. Hoglets grow and lose two sets of baby spines before they get the adult ones they eventually keep.

The hedgehogs are never without spines though, because the baby spines only drop out when the adult ones are fully developed.

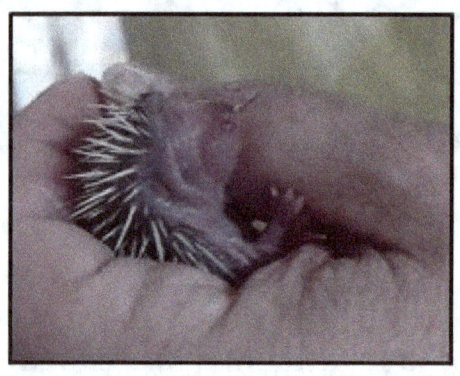

Hedgehogs grow and lose spines all through their lives and as they can have more than 5000 on their backs, that's a lot of spines!

Some people call them spikes or prickles.

Sometimes, they lose a lot at once. This happens when they're stressed, or have parasites, but the spines usually regrow when the hedgehog gets better.

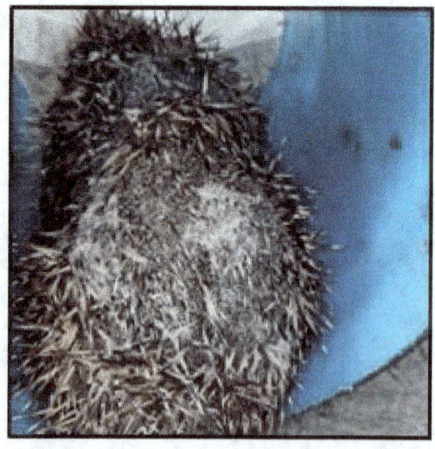

The spines, spikes, or prickles, are made of keratin, which is very strong.

Each one is hollow, has a different marking and ends in a sharp point, so you have to be very careful if you ever pick a hedgehog up.

Heather says you need to scoop one up by putting your hands under either side of its body as if you're carrying a tray.

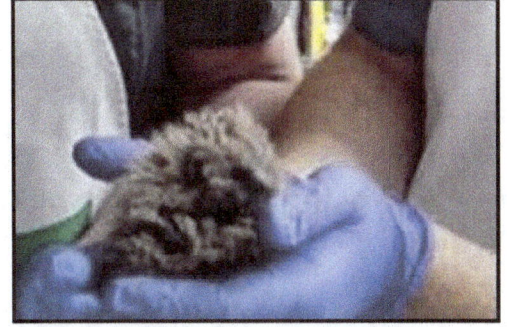

There are no spines on the hedgehog's tummy, but you still have to be careful because they tend to wriggle.

Looking after the hedgehogs is a tiring job.

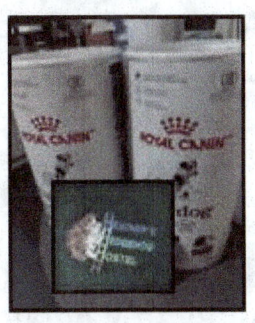

Heather feeds the baby ones every 2 hours with milk from an eye dropper, and to make sure they don't have too much; she puts a special sheath on the end of the dropper with a tiny hole in the end.

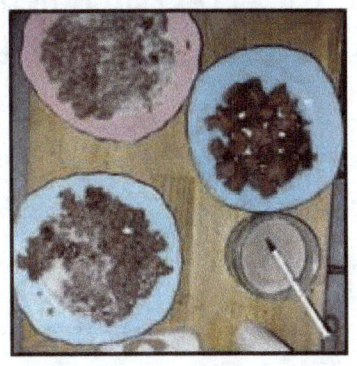

You would usually find them protecting the ends of fishing rods, so Heather is really thinking outside the box!

The milk is actually baby dog milk with some extra additives, but the adult hedgehogs are fed with a combination of different wet and dry cat foods.

Heather doesn't get too attached to her little guests, because once they're better, they go back to where they came from.

As cute as they may be , they're really wild mammals and should be free to roam.

Heather keeps one hedgehog at her hostel as a pet, though.

It's an African Pygmy hedgehog which she got from a rescue centre. It had been abandoned, and Heather has named him Pico.

He is really sweet.

There's a big difference between African Pygmy hedgehogs and the wild kind you find in your garden. African Pygmy hedgehogs are bred in captivity and are kept as pets. They come in different colours and patterns, can grow up to 600g in weight and about 8 inches in length.

They live for about 3 – 6 years, and mainly eat cat or dog food, fruits and vegetables. Although they don't like the cold and need to be kept in a temperature of at least 22 degrees, they don't hibernate.

Heather puts a heat pad in Pico's cage to keep him warm and she also has a hamster wheel in there so he can get a bit of exercise. He runs on it for 8 miles a day!

Our native wild hedgehogs are European hedgehogs. They're much bigger than the African Pygmy type, and are dark brown in colour.

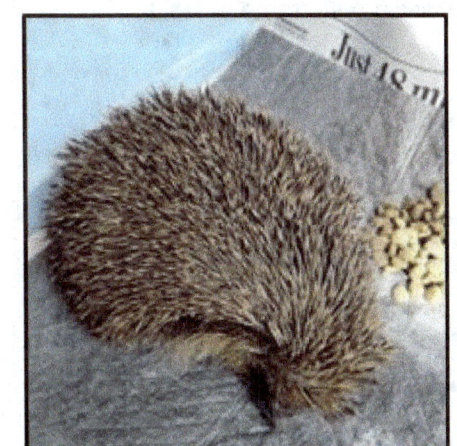

As they get older, these hedgehogs turn more of a golden brown, which is how you can tell their age.

They can grow up to 1.5 kg in weight and about 14 inches in length.

They usually live for about 2 to 3 years and in the wild they eat creepie crawlies, like beetles, caterpillars, earwigs, earthworms, fly larvae, millipedes and slugs.

They hibernate in winter.

Some people build hedgehog homes in their gardens so these endangered creatures have somewhere safe to shelter, hibernate and raise their hoglets.

They can be built at any time of year, but aren't usually used until the weather turns and the hedgehogs are looking for somewhere to hibernate.

Hedgehog homes need to have quite a large main chamber so the creature can give birth to its babies, and turn around and walk in and out, but the entrance corridor needs to be narrow so badgers, dogs and other larger predators can't get inside.

They're usually boxes made of wood with a roof.

Some people use corrugated material for the roof and put a narrow drainpipe through it for ventilation. It needs to be screwed down so it doesn't get knocked off.

Often these homes are covered with leaves and woody garden cuttings to insulate them from the cold and heat, but you have to make sure the ventilation pipe and entrance remain clear.

Ideally, hedgehog homes should be lined with a layer of small dead, dry leaves, and placed it in a quiet part of the garden where vegetation is thick, or behind a shed out of the wind.

They should be cleaned out every year.

This can be done either by unscrewing the roof, or lifting the whole box up ... but obviously not when the hedgehogs are inside!

You can check this by putting something in front of the entrance of the hedgehog home that won't blow away, but can be easily moved by a hedgehog. A scrunched-up piece of newspaper is ideal.

If it's in a different place when you check the next morning, you'll know your little guests are still around.

When the hedgehogs come into the hostel, Heather makes a note of the date, where they were found and

the contact details of the person who brought them in.

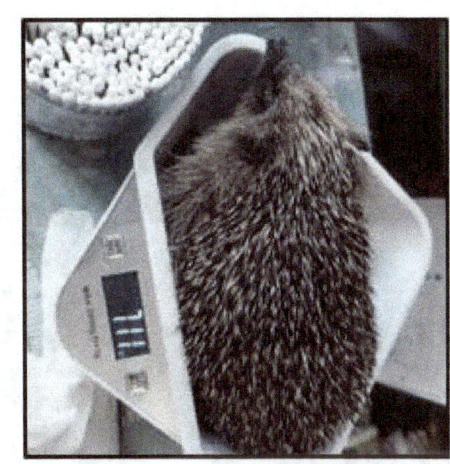

She finds out what's wrong with them, weighs them, cleans them up and makes sure they all have a cosy bed to sleep in.

Heather gives them lots of love and attention, and they all have names.

Sometimes, the person who brings the hedgehogs in has already named the little creatures, but if not, Heather chooses something suitable.

She says she can tell them apart because they all have different markings on their spines and their cute, bright eyed, faces are all unique.

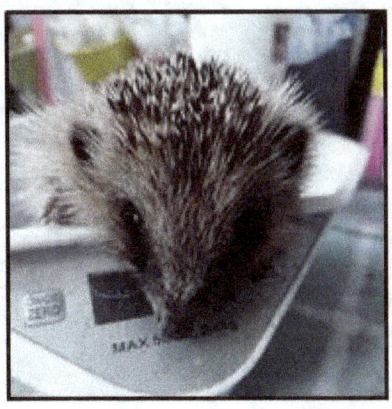

She monitors their progress every day and when the little creatures are better, Heather contacts the person who brought them in to come and take them back to where they found them.

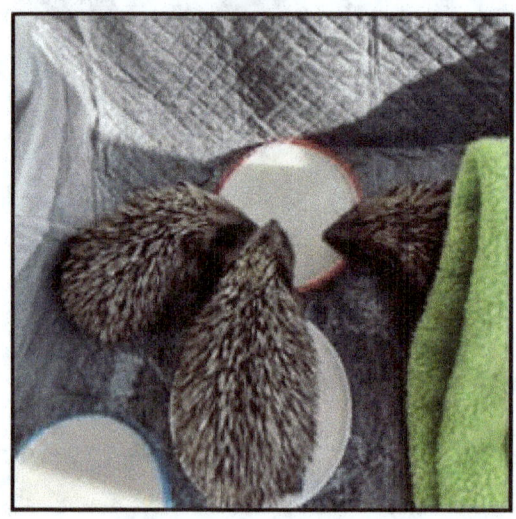

In the hostel the baby hedgehogs are fed on milk and special food which Heather mixes up, but in the wild, they love munching on insects like beetles and worms, and also enjoy eating fruits and vegetables.

Hedgehogs can't see very well, but have good hearing and a great sense of smell. They can find their food even in the dark.

It's like they have a special superpower and often you'll hear them snuffling around at night as they forage for food.

They're very noisy!

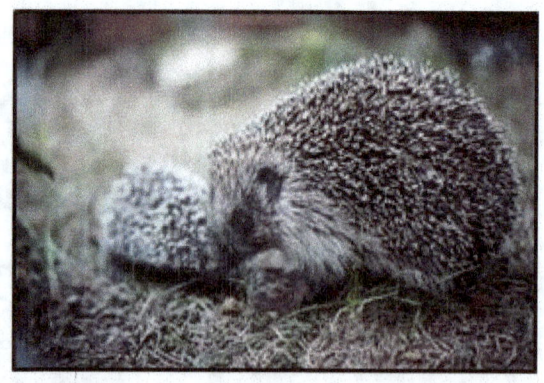

If you see one in your garden and want to give it a meal, make sure to only give it food and water in a shallow dish .

Please don't give it milk, because that will upset his stomach and the hedgehog may die of dehydration.

Some of the hedgehogs taken to the hostel need medical help and Heather gives them special medicine to make them better.

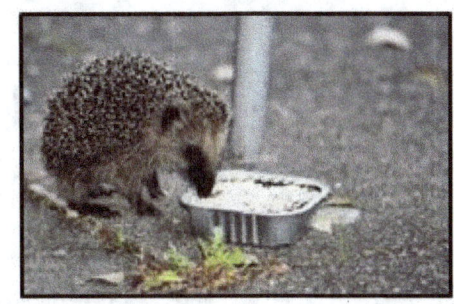

She also gives them a bath and gets rid of any fleas they might have.

Some people think all hedgehogs have fleas but that's not true. They only get them if they're ill.

Heather baths the hedgehogs in the sink and gently pats them dry with a towel.

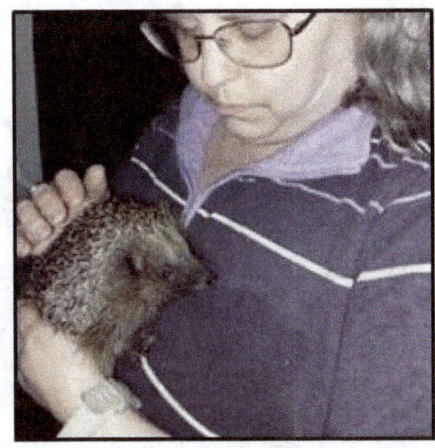

Then, she'll cup them in her hands, hold them close to her body and stroke their prickles.

She makes sure to stroke backwards and not forwards, just like you would if you were stroking a cat or a dog.

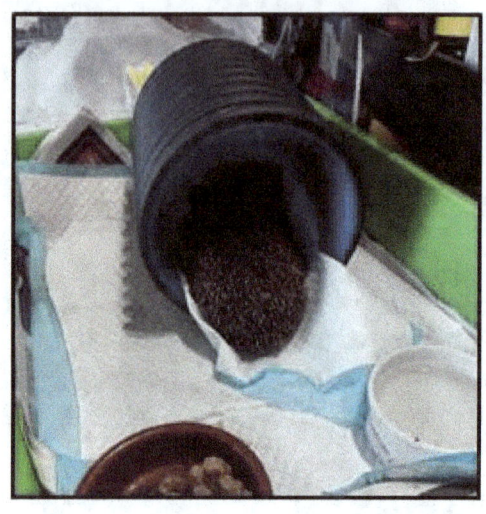

Hedgehogs. can actually move very fast and like to explore, so Heather keeps them all in their own pet boxes.

She lines the bottoms with paper to make it easier to clear up after they've been to the toilet and finished feeding.

The really poorly ones have a box to themselves, but depending on why they are at the hostel, some of the others can share.

Gary, the huge hedgehog that had been used as a football recovered in a rabbit hutch outside. He was too big to go in the boxes indoors.

Now, you might wonder how Gary had survived the kicking, and that's because hedgehog spines protect them from blows and falls.

You see. each hedgehog spine has a very sharp point at one end, and although it's very hard, it can flex and bend.

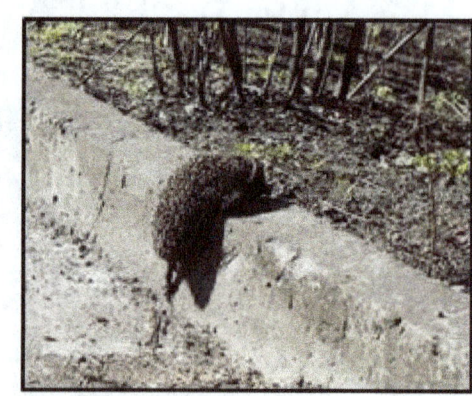

The other end of the spine goes inside the hedgehog's skin, but it has a round bulb type root, so it can't be pushed into the creature's flesh.

That's probably just as well as hedgehogs can climb!

They've been known to throw themselves through the air from great heights and still be fine when they've landed on the ground.

Yes, the hedgehog spines are very useful. Not only do they protect them from predators, but also help them swim and float in water.

Their spines are hollow, air filled tubes, so when these spiny mammals get tired of swimming, they can roll over on their backs and float like boats!

In case you're wondering why hedgehogs swim, it's so they can reach any food they smell either in, or, on, the other side of a stretch of water.

Also, the water offers them a drink if they're thirsty, but as they usually only venture out at night to forage for food, it's unlikely you'll see these nocturnal mammals swimming.

Although, they're good swimmers, hedgehogs sometimes drown in garden ponds or swimming pools .

That's because they can get into the water easily, but can't always get out.

Often the walls are just too steep.

One of the fascinating things about hedgehogs is the way they curl up into a ball when they need extra protection from the cold, or predators.

If they feel a bit uncomfortable, but aren't sure if they're in danger, they bristle their spines so they point outwards.

Then they pull their head, back legs and tail in so the spines cover all the areas where there isn't any protection

It's like being sheltered by a spiky umbrella, but means they can run away if they need to.

When the danger is more serious, they curl up into a full ball by tightening up all the muscles round the body where the spines meet the fur.

It's a bit like pulling a drawstring on a spikey bag and all the vulnerable bits get safely tucked up inside.

They can stay that way for hours!

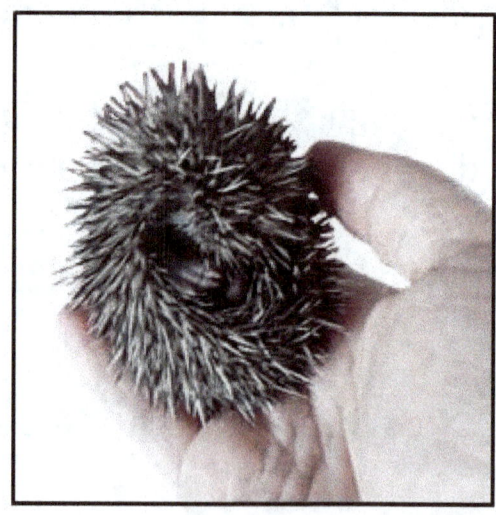

As clever as they are, these unique little creatures are on the decline.

In the UK, hedgehogs are found in woodland edges, hedges, farmland, parks, and gardens.

They like to wander, but now a lot of people fence in their gardens, so the hedgehogs can't move around so easily to find food.

Another problem facing hedgehogs is the use of garden netting. That's because of their spines.

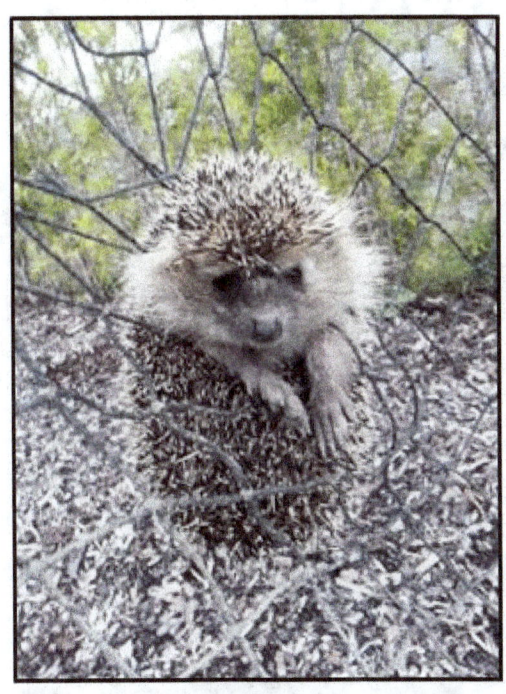

Hedgehogs can flatten them to crawl into tight spaces, but unless they can get straight out the other side, the spines often pin them in place and they get stuck.

Also, many get run over on the roads, cut by lawnmowers and strimmers, poisoned by garden chemicals, or accidentally burned in bonfires.

It's sad!

Like all animals, hedgehogs need food to survive, but as the weather gets colder, the food they eat gets harder to find.

That's why they fatten themselves up as much as possible on things like beetles, caterpillars, worms, slugs and snails, during the warmer months so they can hibernate in the Winter.

Hedgehogs build shelters in which to hibernate out of dead leaves, twigs and feathers, but sometimes you'll find them hiding in piles of logs, compost heaps, or under garden sheds.

They don't often come out during the day, but you'll hear them snuffling and grunting at night when they're searching for food.

The little things need to build up their fat reserves to see them through the cold, winter months between November and March.

When they hibernate, hedgehogs go to sleep for several months to save energy. They do this by dropping their heart rate right down from 190 beats per minute to 20, and almost stop breathing.

It's the only way the little animals can go so many months without food, and unless they wake up because the temperature drops so low they're in danger of freezing to death, you won't see, or hear them again until Spring.

Hedgehogs help out in the garden, because they feed on all the insects that attack your vegetables, but the species is disappearing.

Their world is full of danger, and much of it is caused by man.

If you see one on the road, don't run over it. Thousands are killed by vehicles every year.

Help it cross the road safely and find a field or den to rest in.

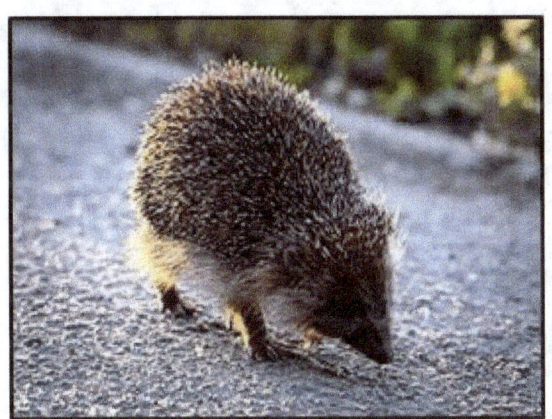

You can help look after the hedgehogs in your area by leaving food out and giving them some water and shelter when it's hot.

Hedgehogs happily eat food left outside in your garden, and use it to supplement, rather than replace their natural diet.

The best foods to provide for them are, meat-based cat or dog food, specially-made hedgehog food, and cat biscuits.

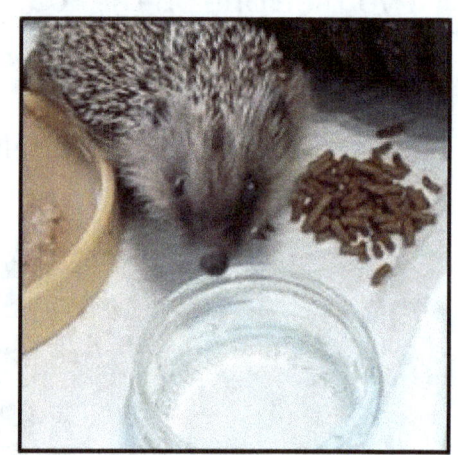

Hedgehogs suffer in hot weather and if you see one out in the day it won't be sunbathing.

It may be in need of immediate attention.

Here are some simple things you can do to help.

🦔 Put out water in shallow dishes for them. It could be a lifeline.

🦔 Create cool and shaded areas in your garden to offer hedgehogs and other wildlife somewhere to escape the heat.

🦔 Check for hedgehogs in long grass and overgrown areas before mowing or strimming the grass to prevent any harm or injuries.

As you can see, Heather is a very kind lady and really looks after the little hedgehogs. Her hedgehog hostel is now a registered charity so she can accept donations.

Everything is appreciated, especially old newspapers and baby dog food, but it would be really nice if Heather had some more volunteers to help her with her important work.

Obviously, not everyone lives near Chatteris, but now you know a bit more about these adorable little mammals, perhaps you could look out for them where you live?

Don't forget to check your gardens, you never know where they might be hiding!

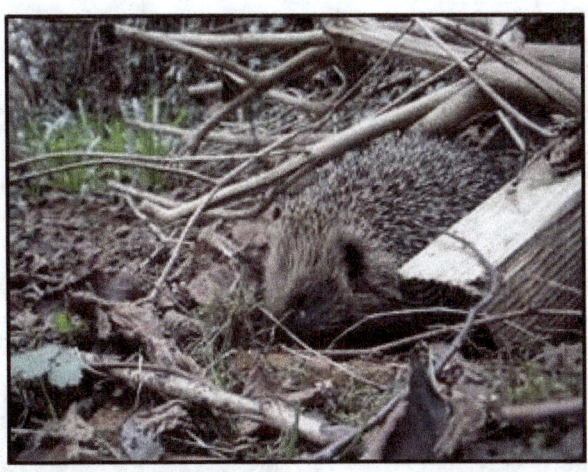

What is a hedgehog's most unique feature?

Answer: A hedgehog's most unique feature is its prickly quills that help protect it from predators. On average, a hedgehog has about 5,000 to 7,000 spikes covering its back and sides.

When do hedgehogs usually come out to explore?

Answer: Hedgehogs are mostly nocturnal, so they come out to explore and search for food at night.

How do hedgehogs protect themselves from danger?

Answer: When they feel threatened, hedgehogs curl up into a tight ball, covering their soft belly with their spiky quills for protection.

What do hedgehogs like to eat?

Answer: Hedgehogs are insectivores, and they enjoy feasting on insects, snails, worms, and sometimes even fruits.

Where do hedgehogs sleep during the daytime?

Answer: Hedgehogs build cosy nests in burrows, piles of leaves, or under bushes to sleep during the daytime.

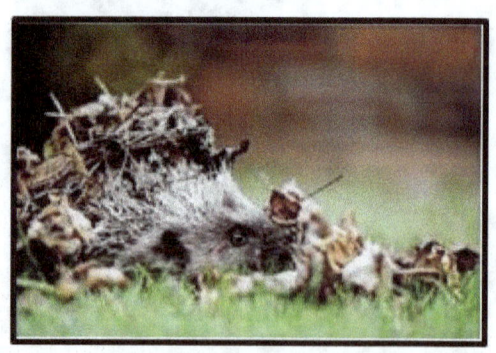

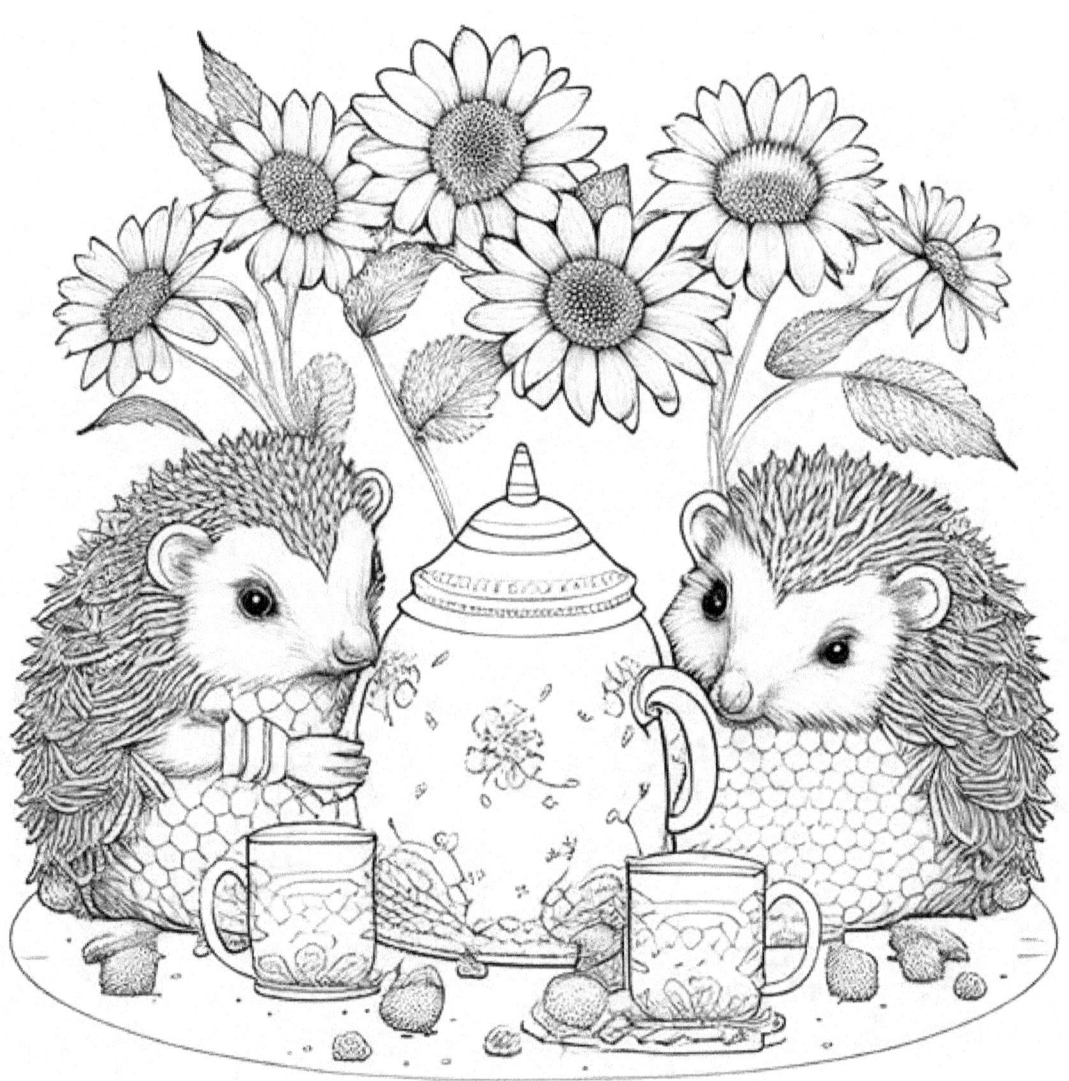

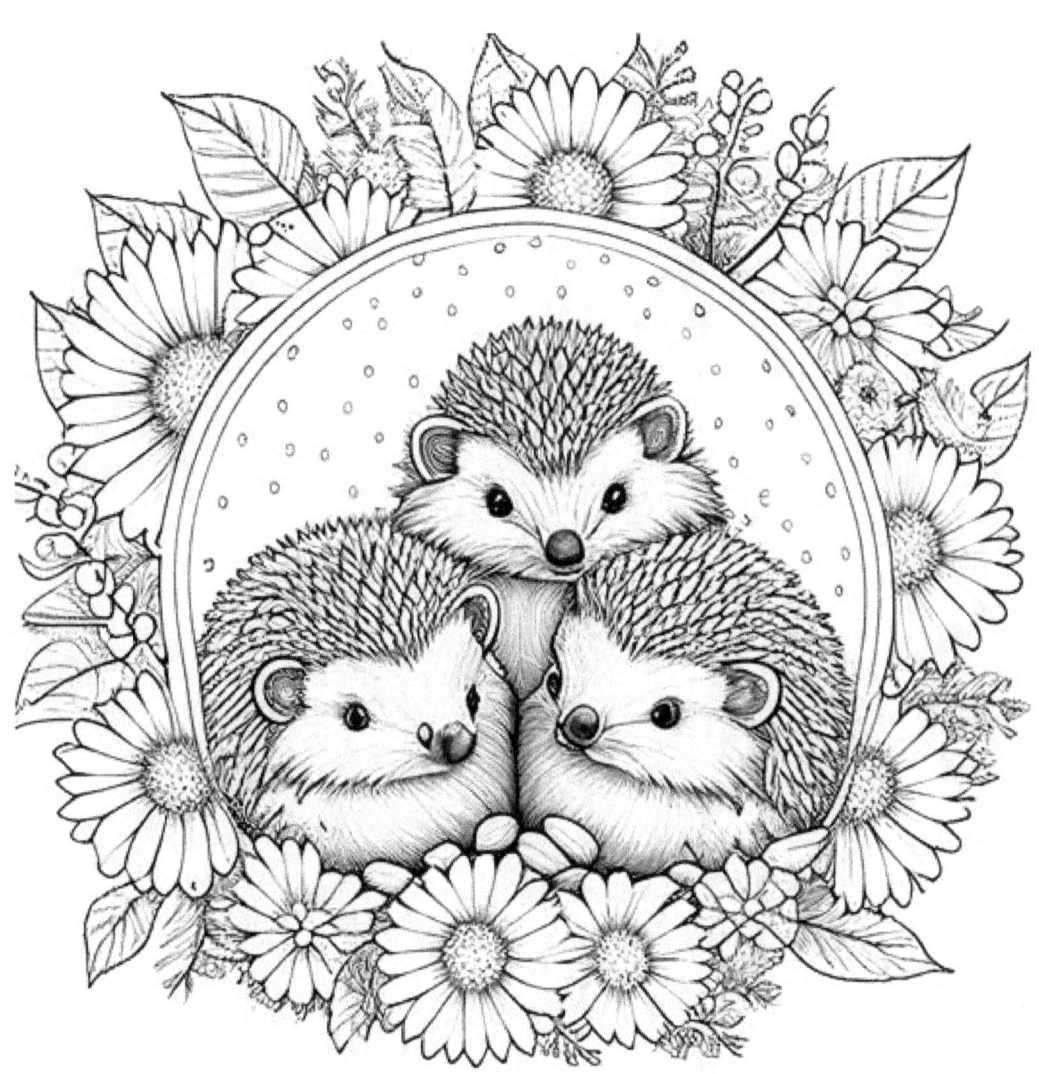

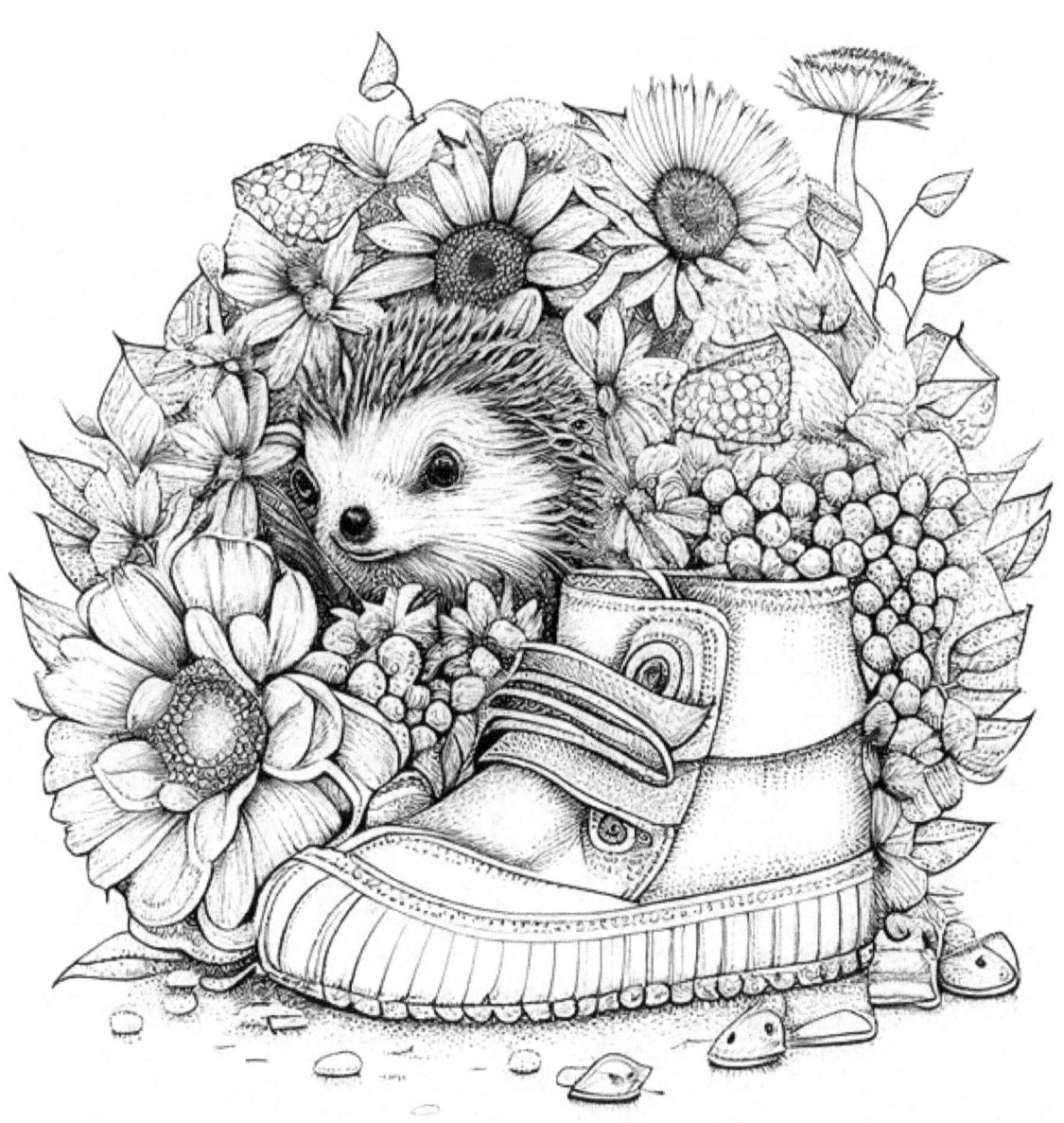

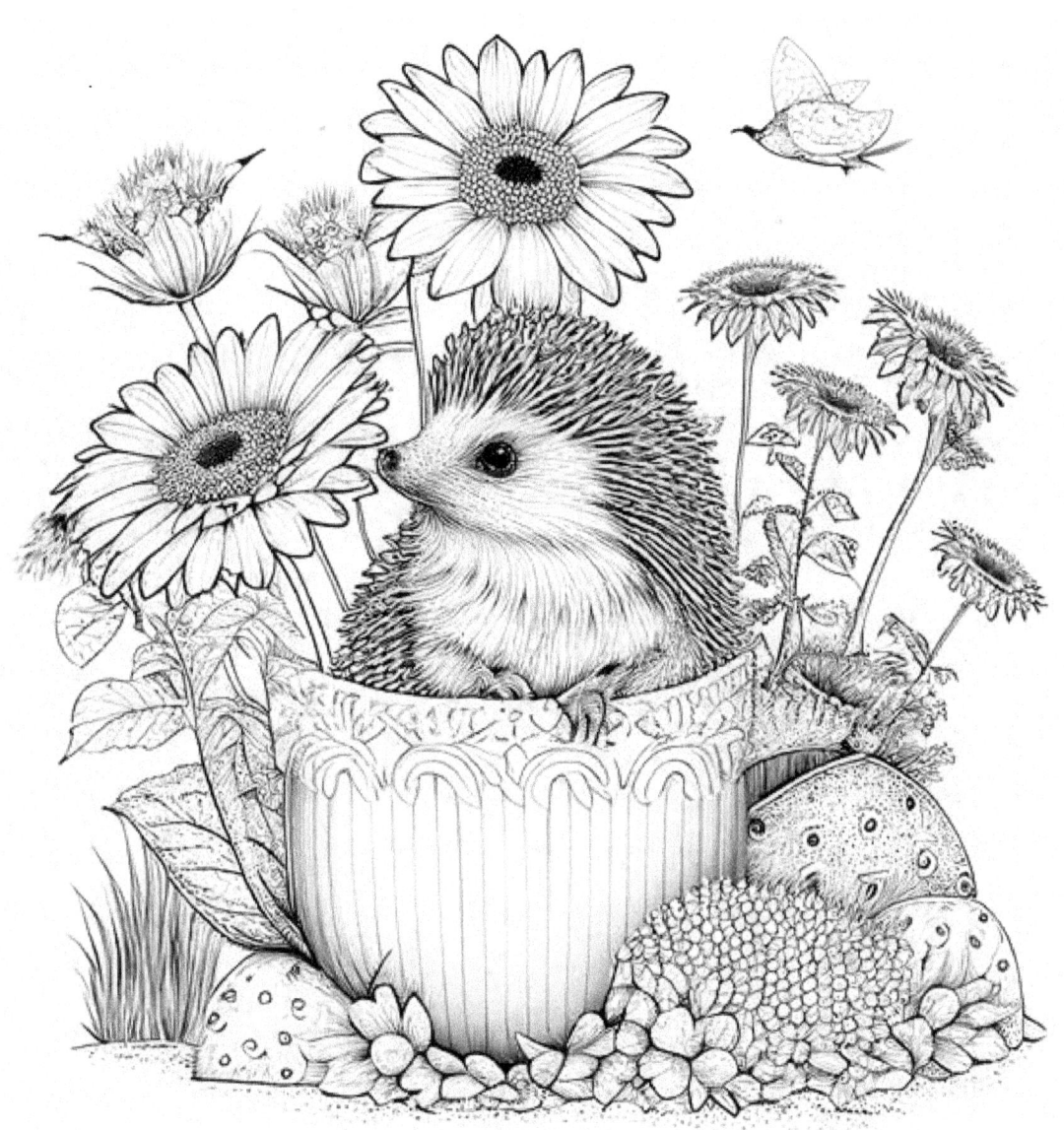

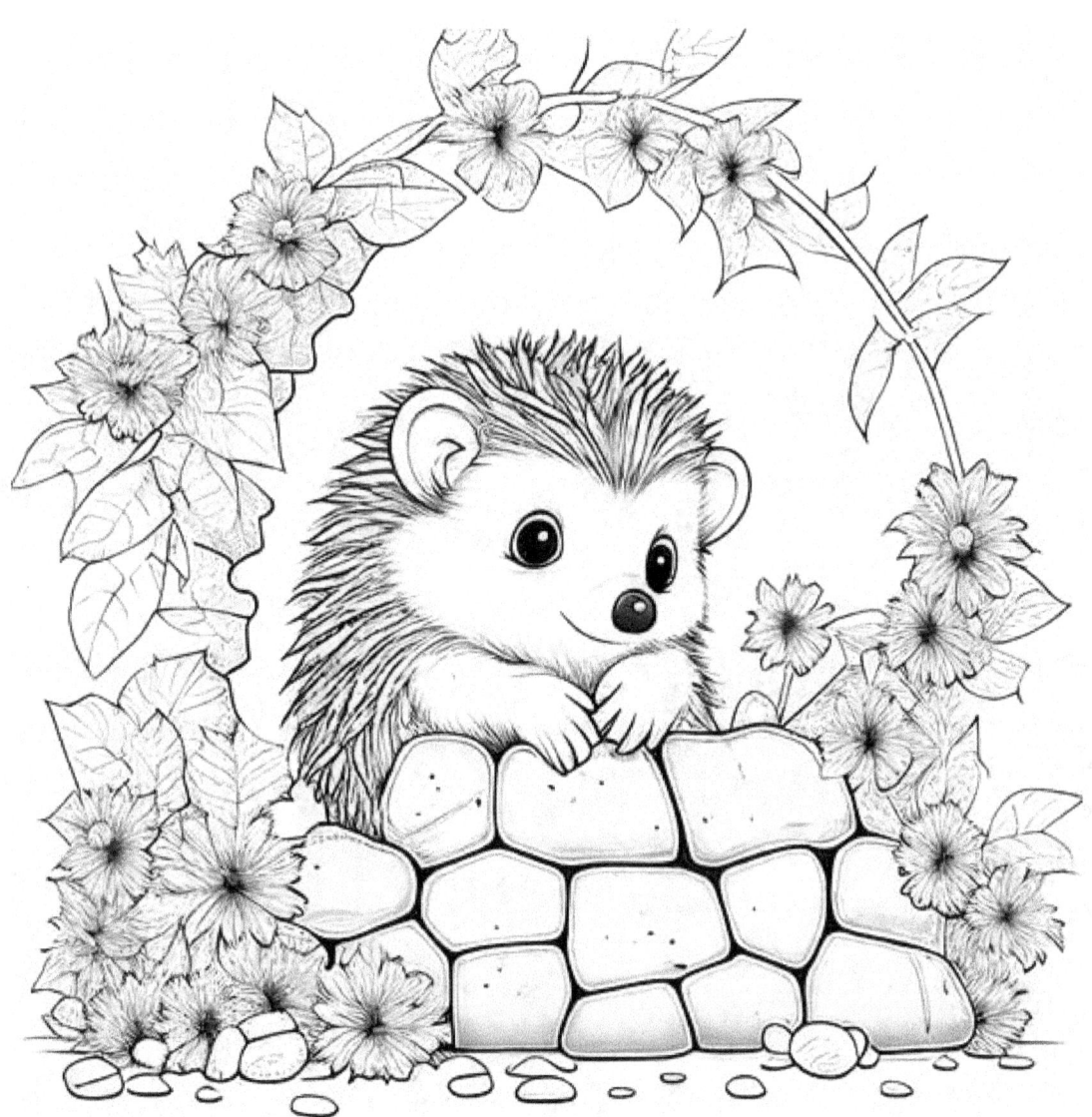

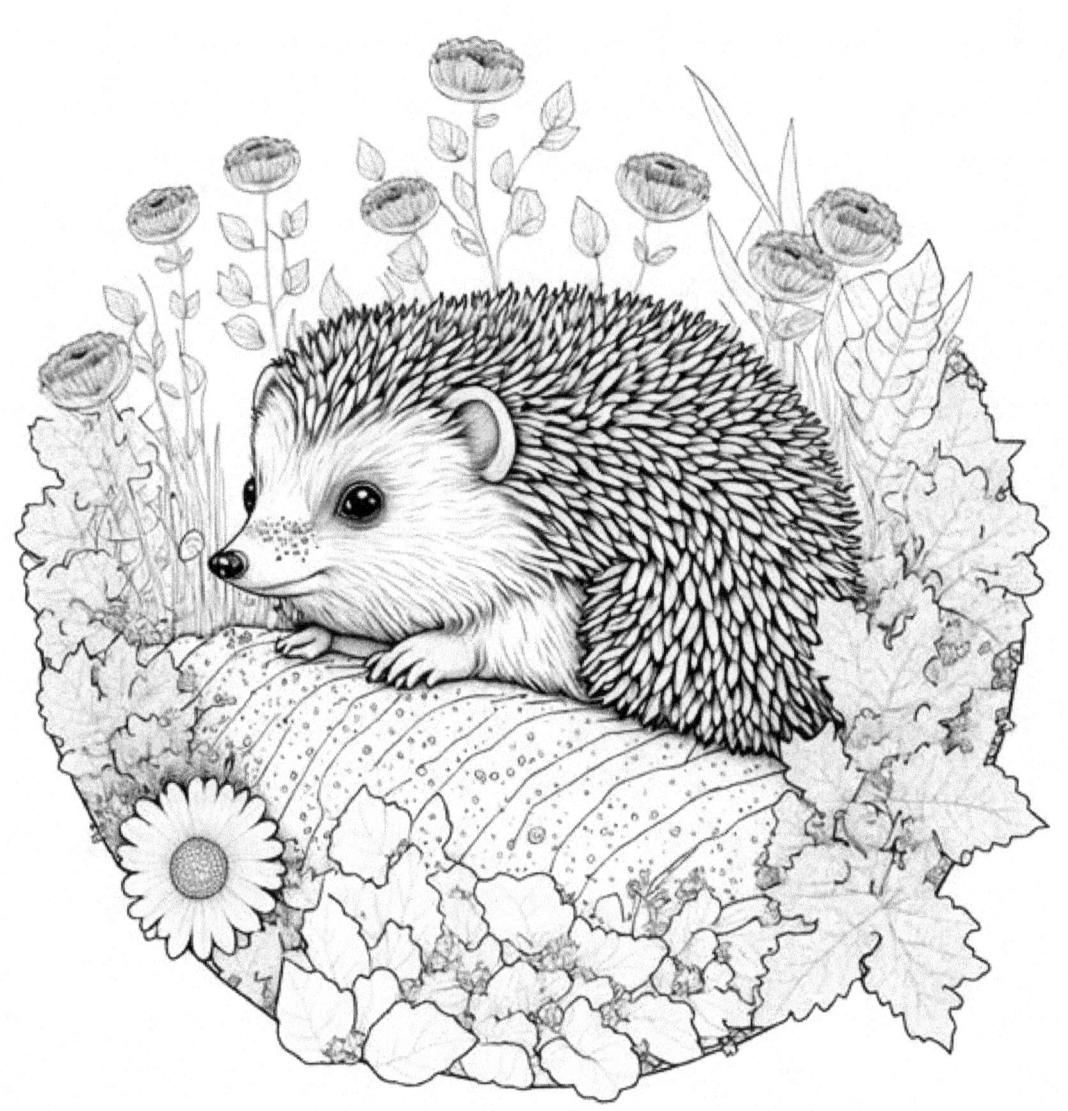

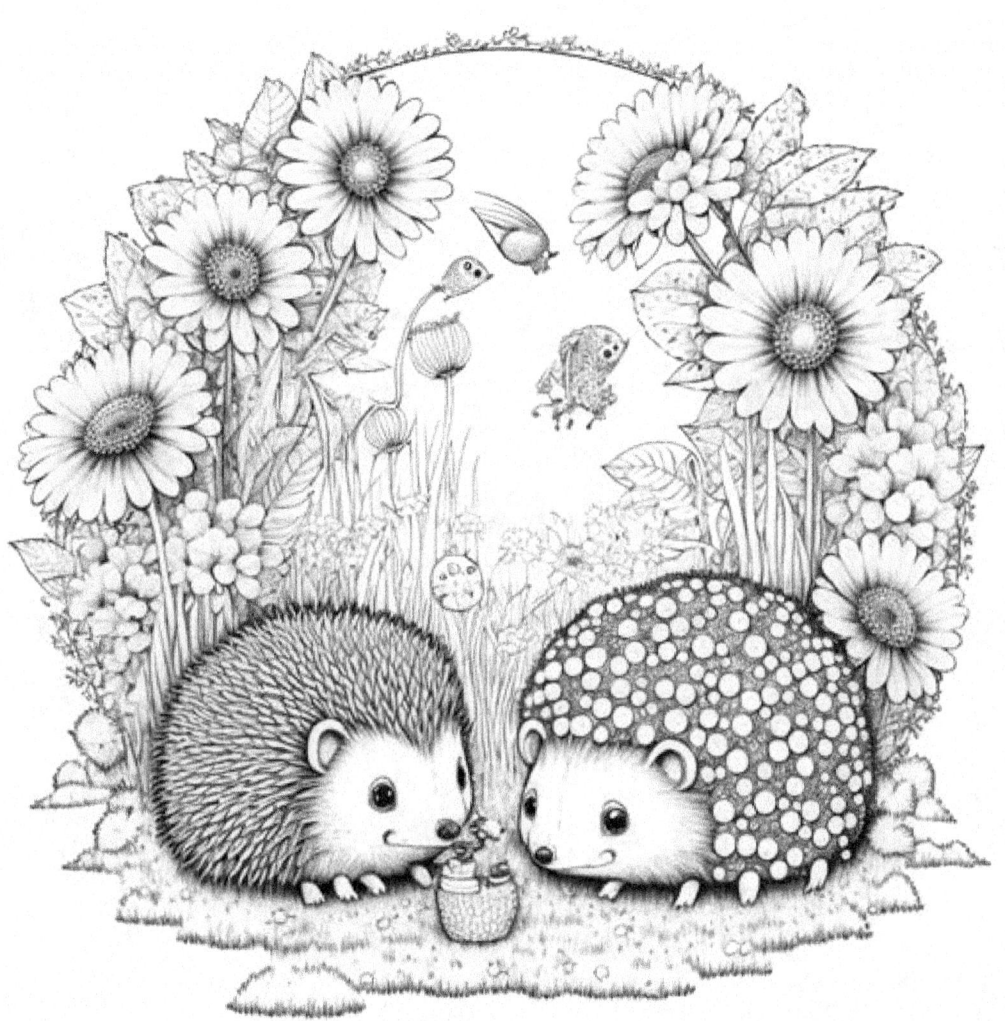

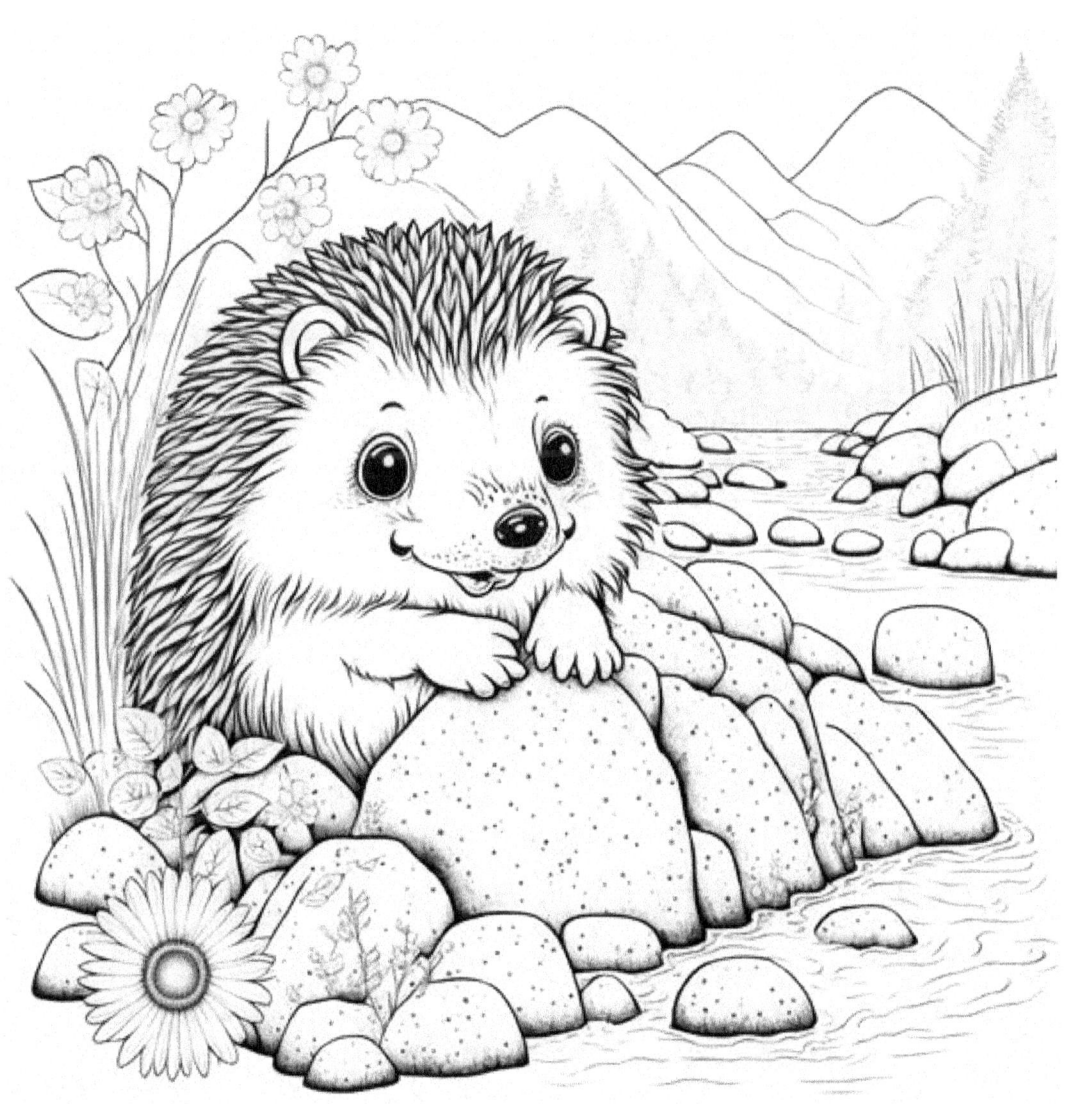

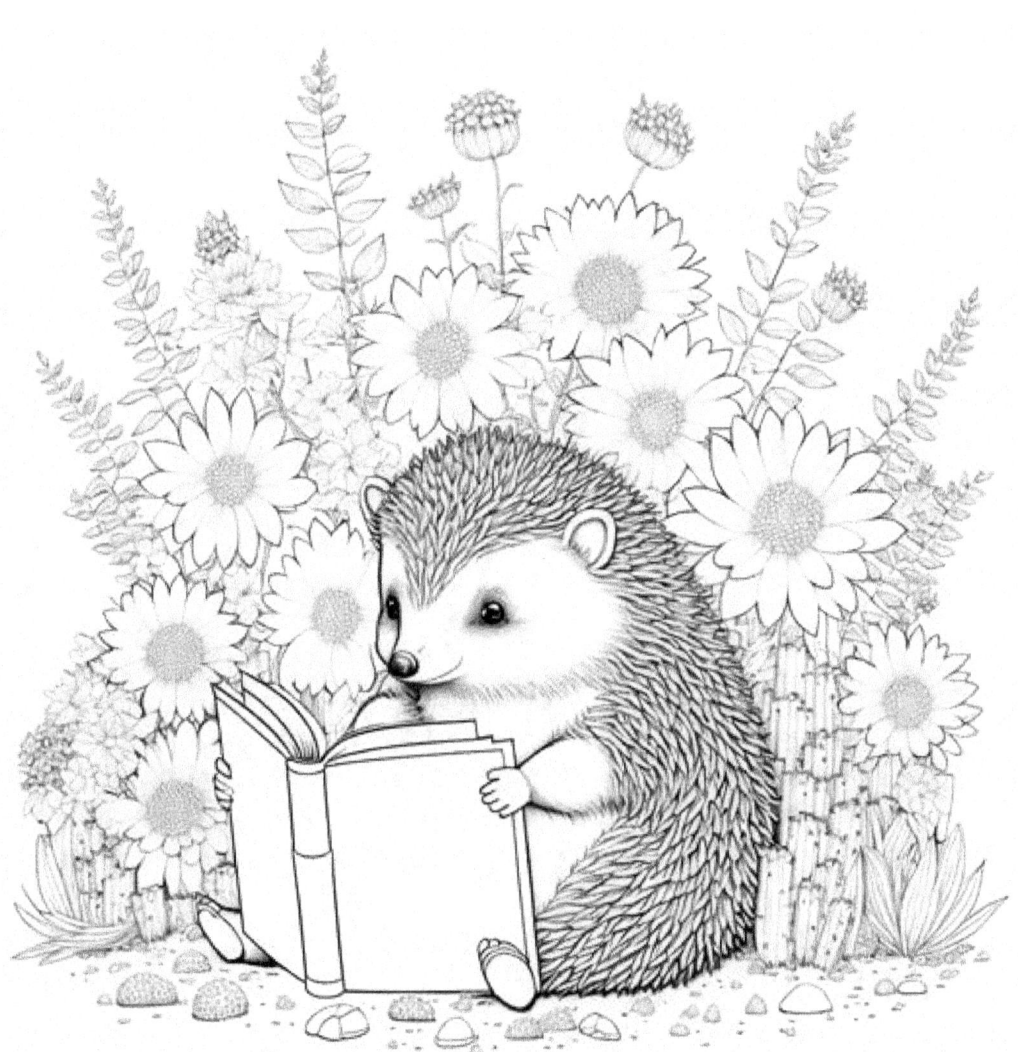

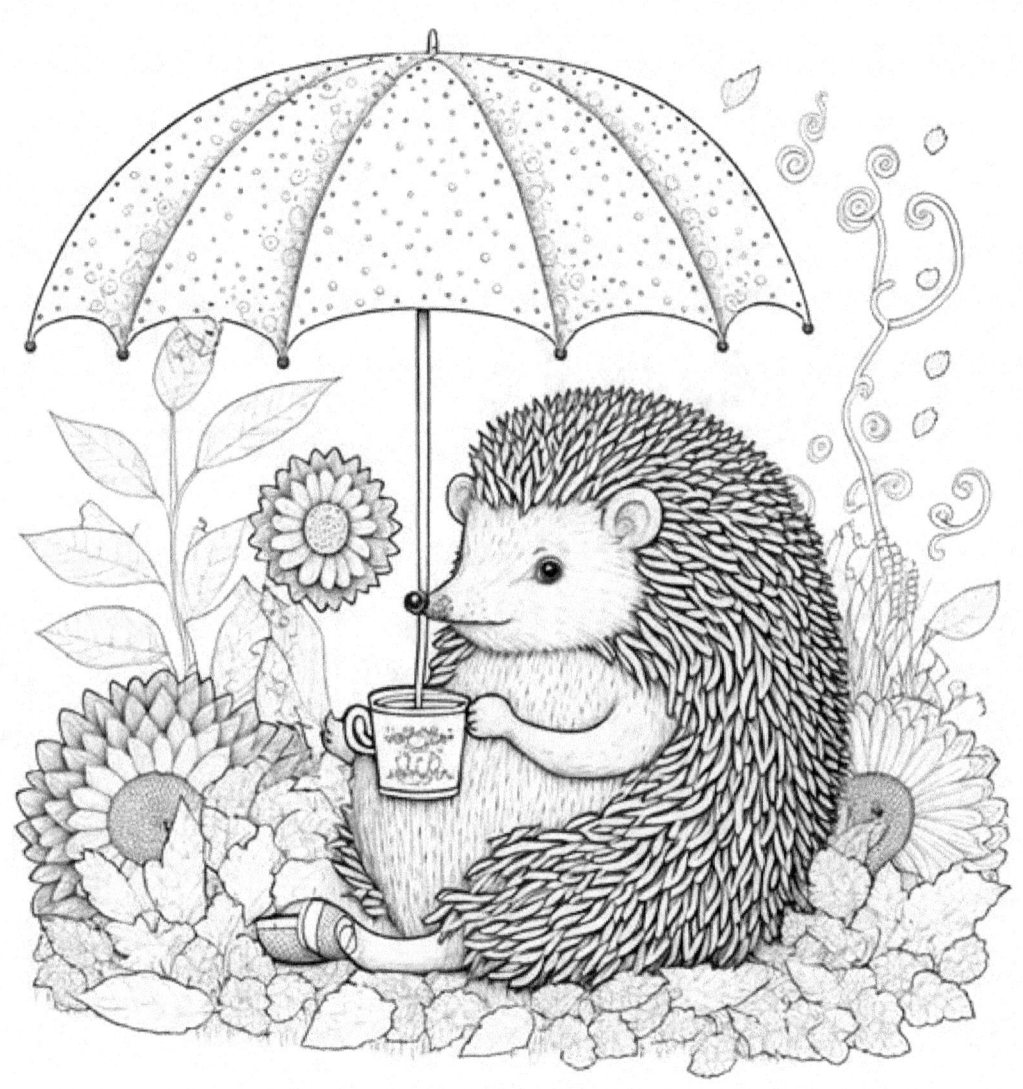

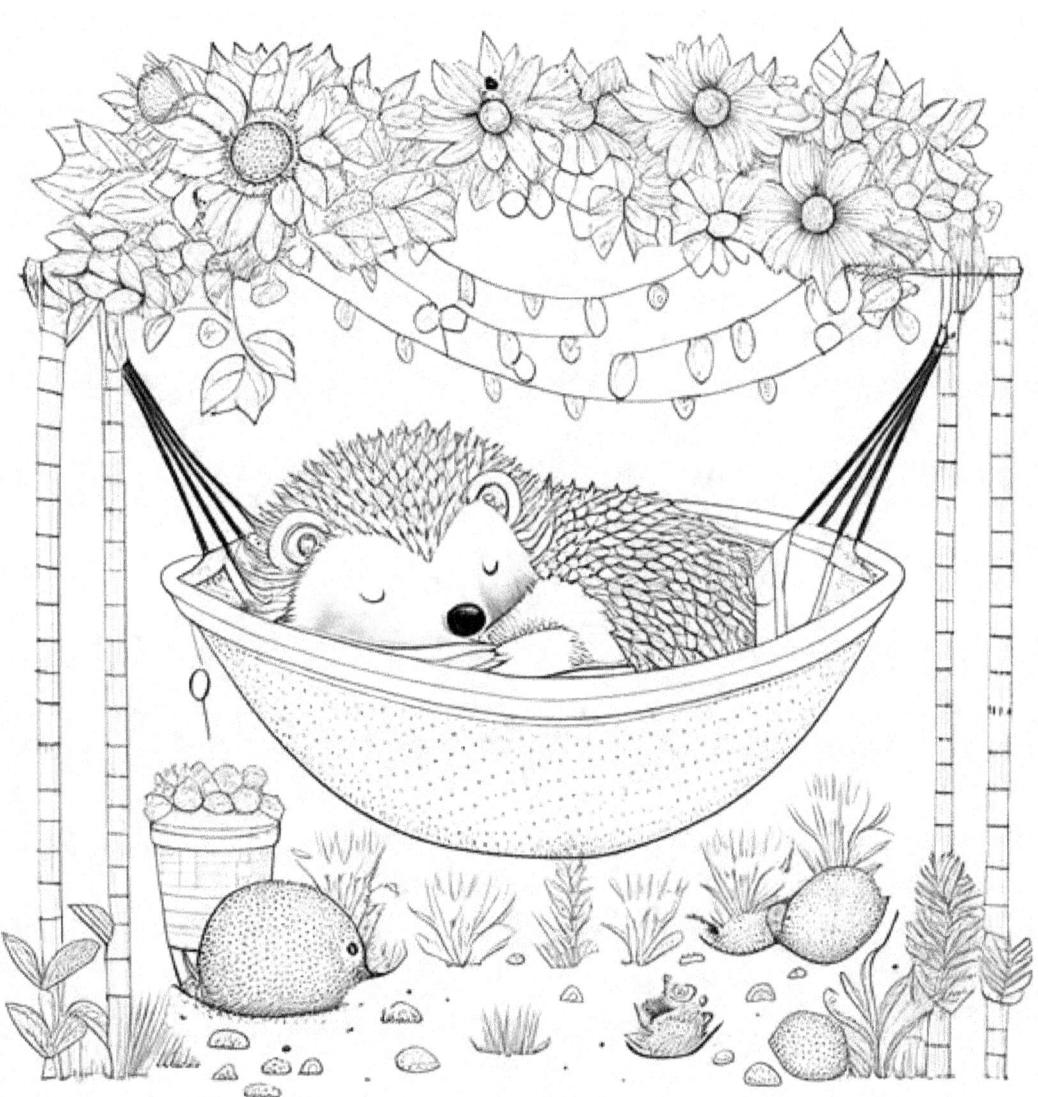

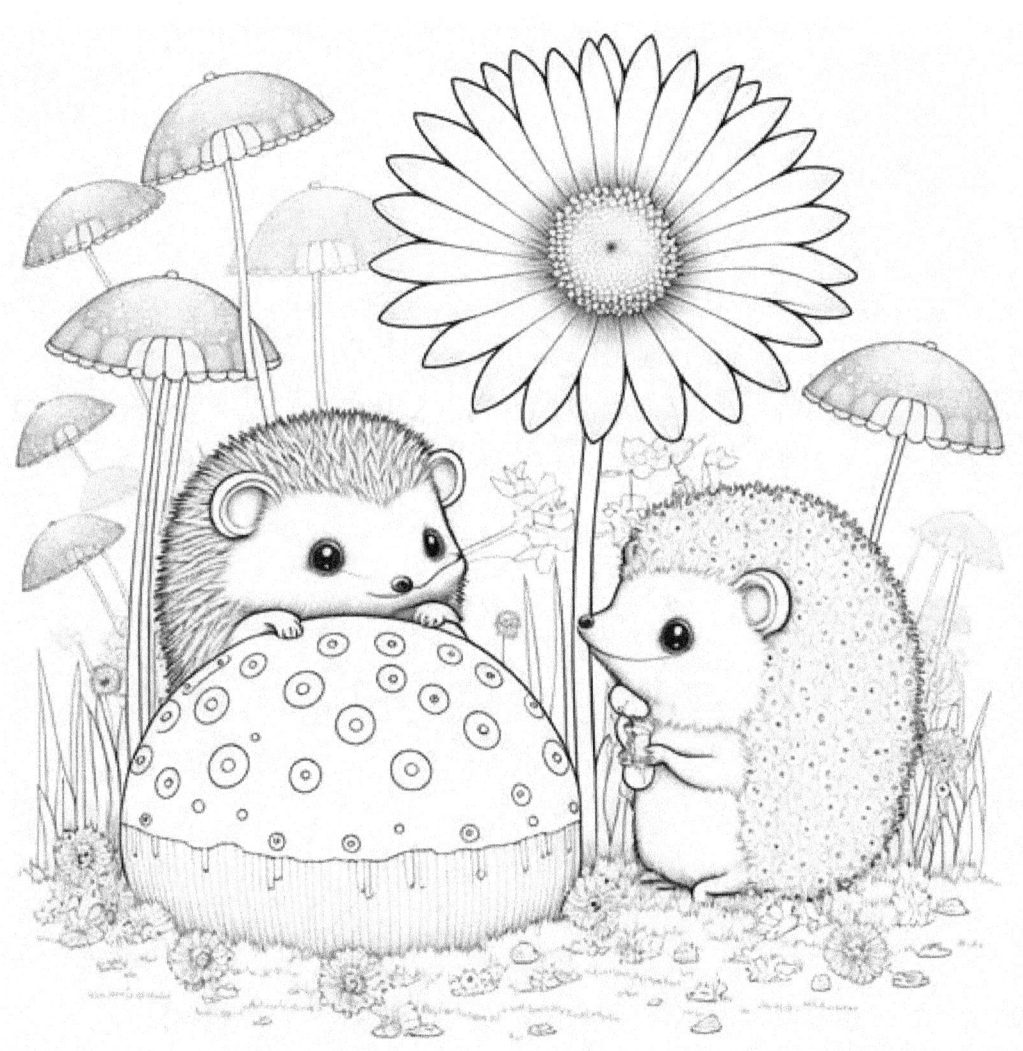

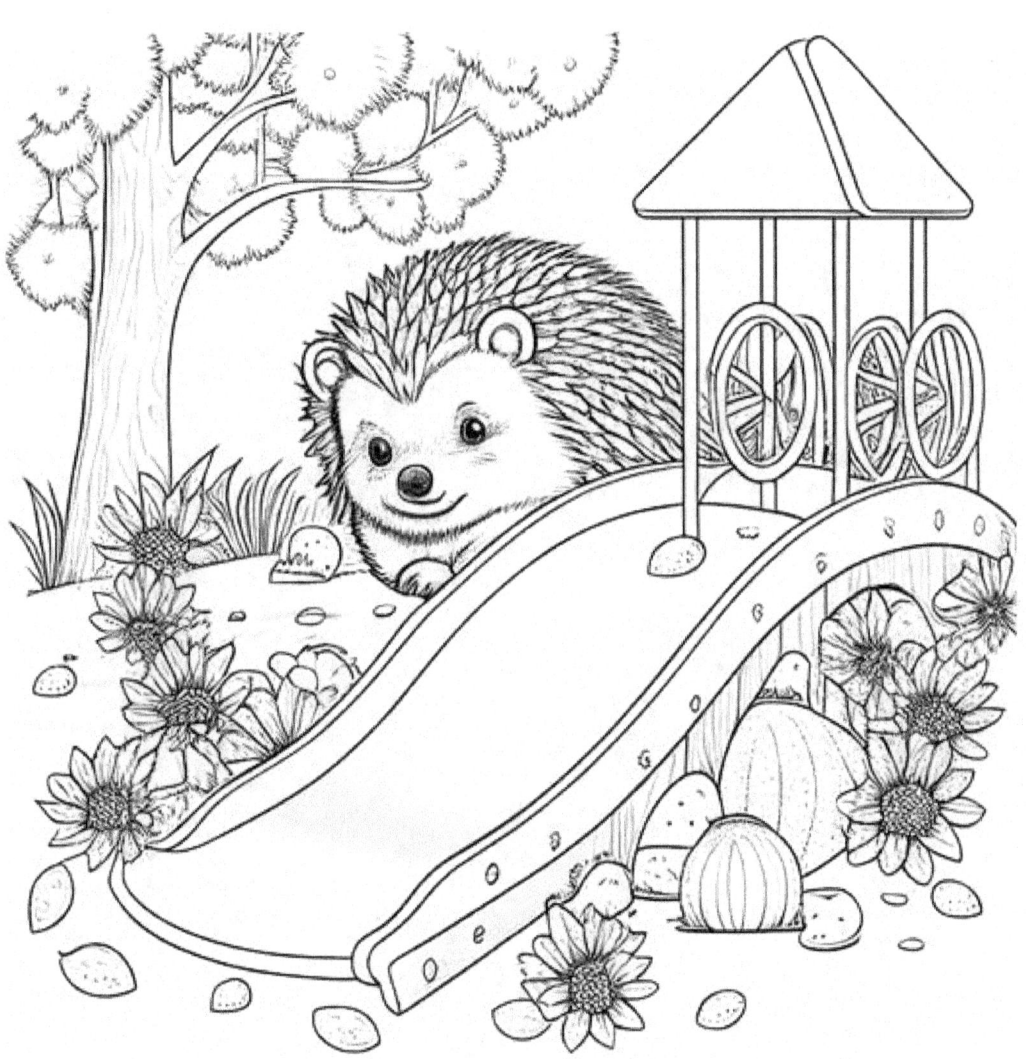

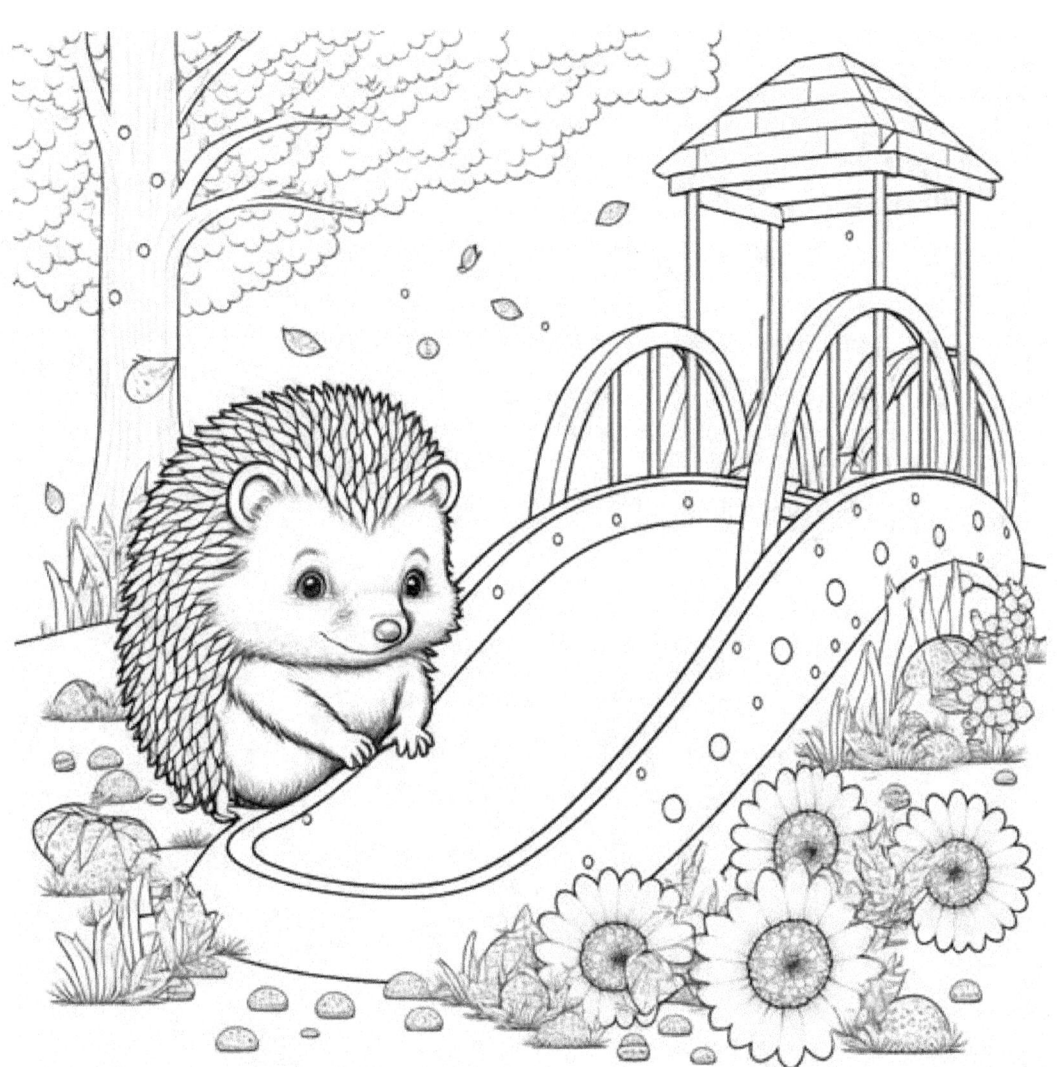

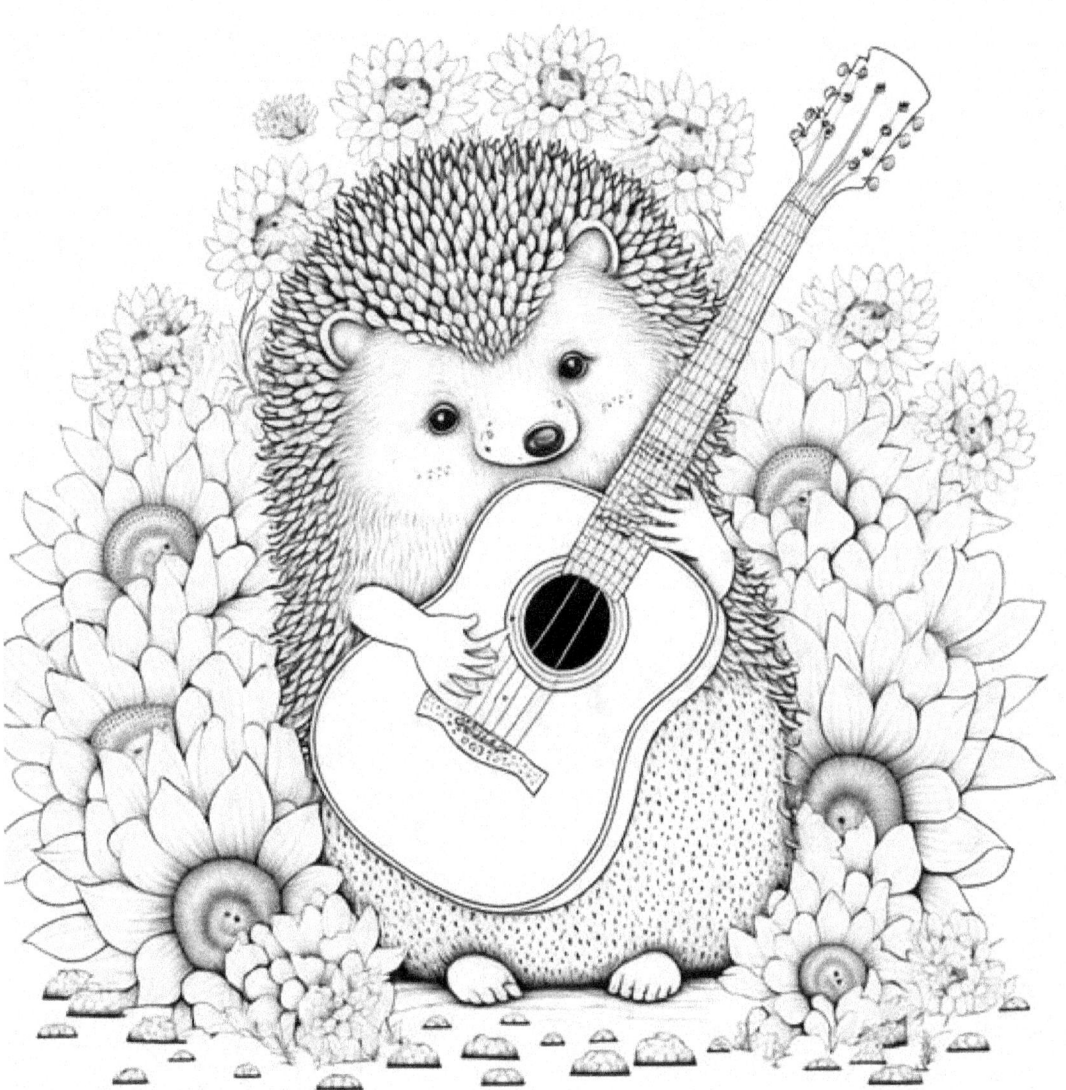

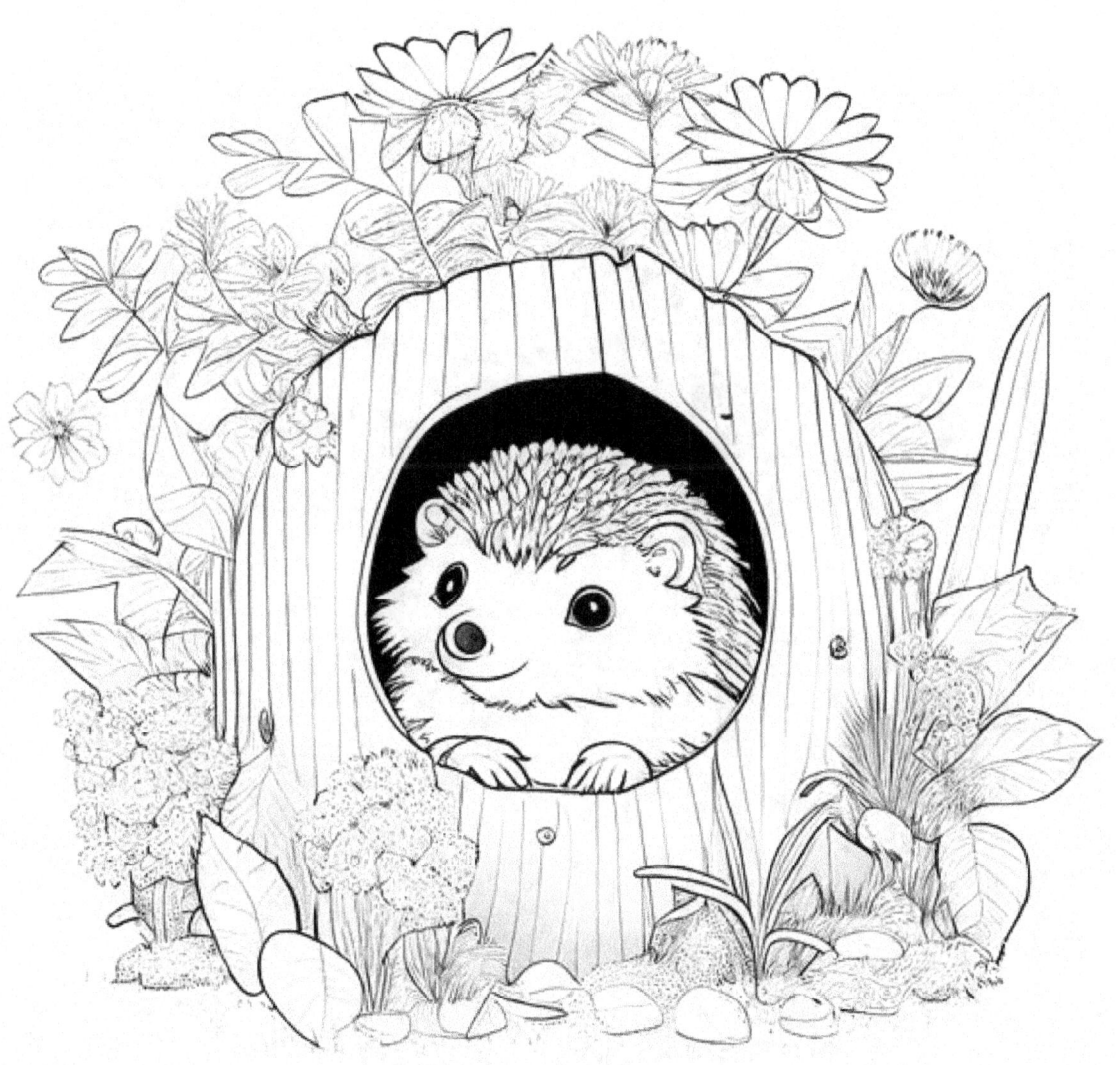

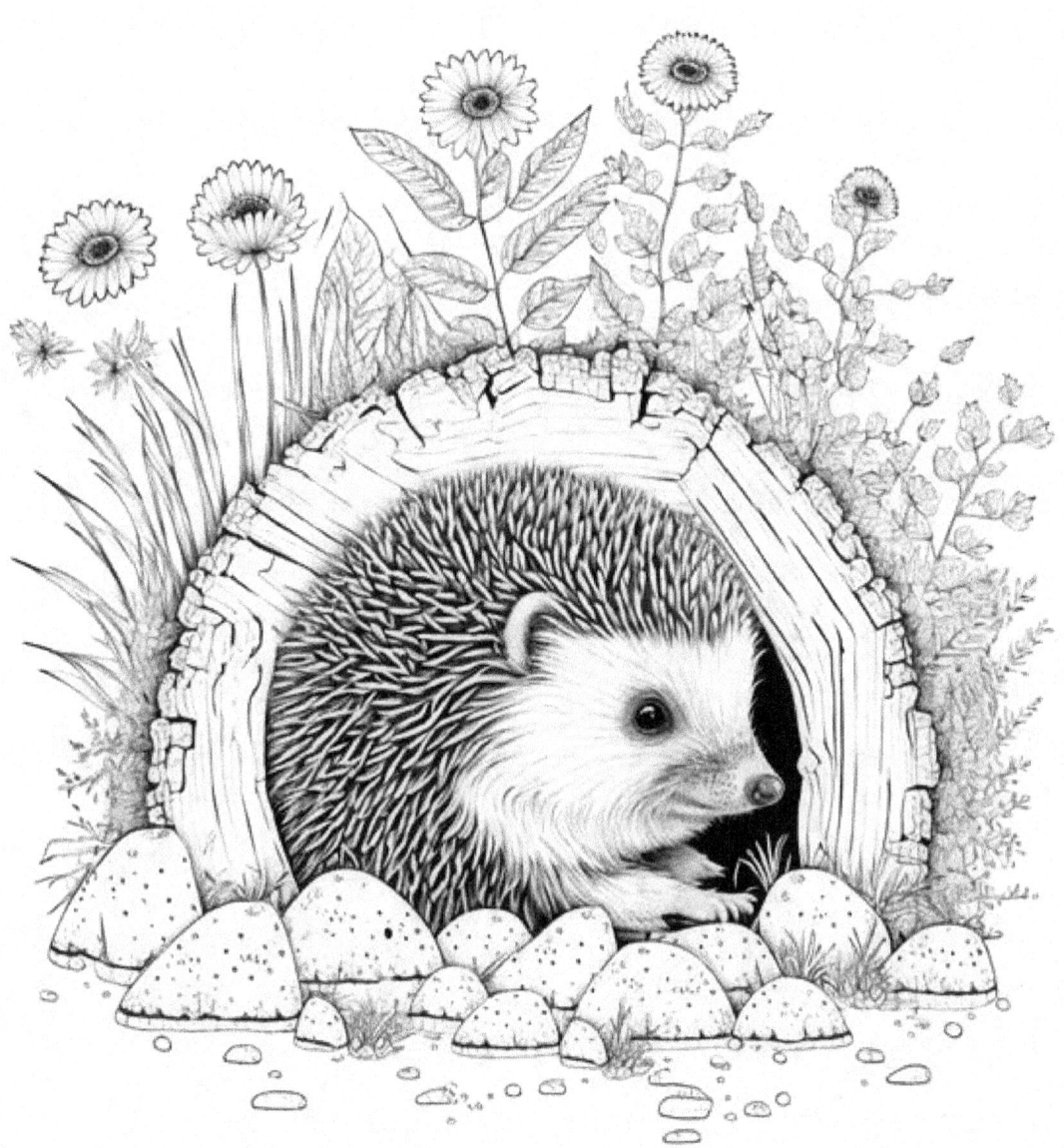

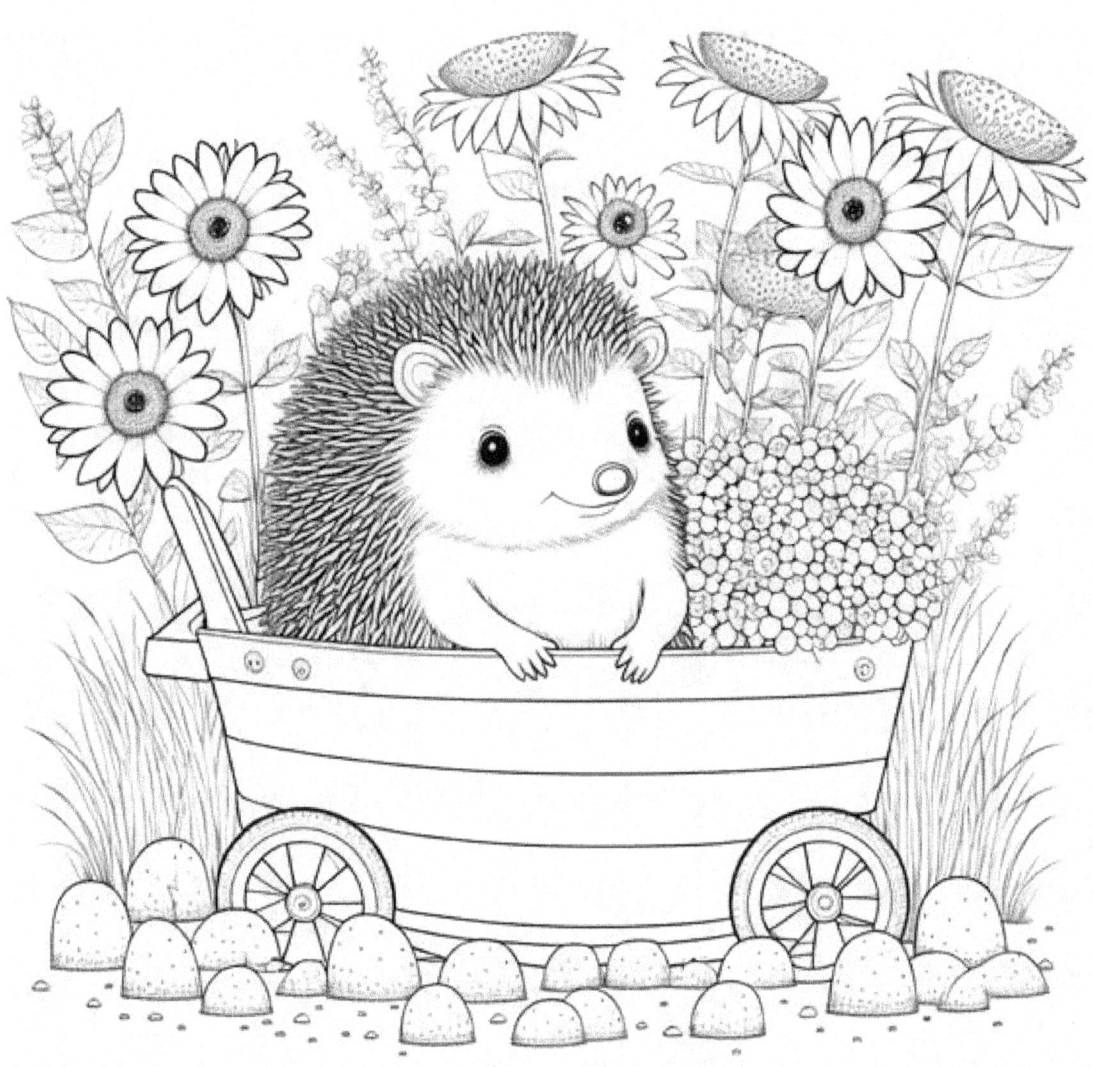

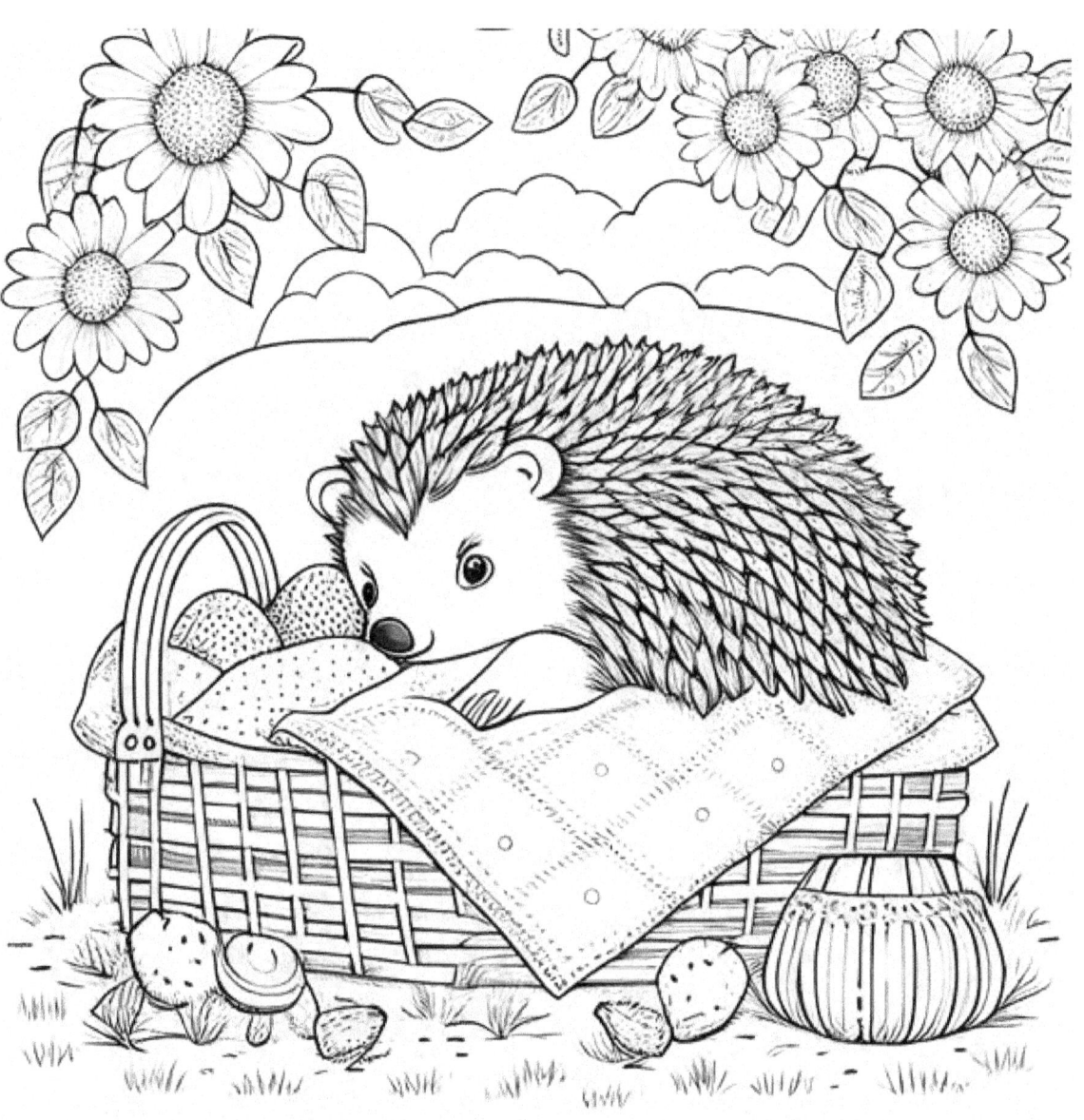

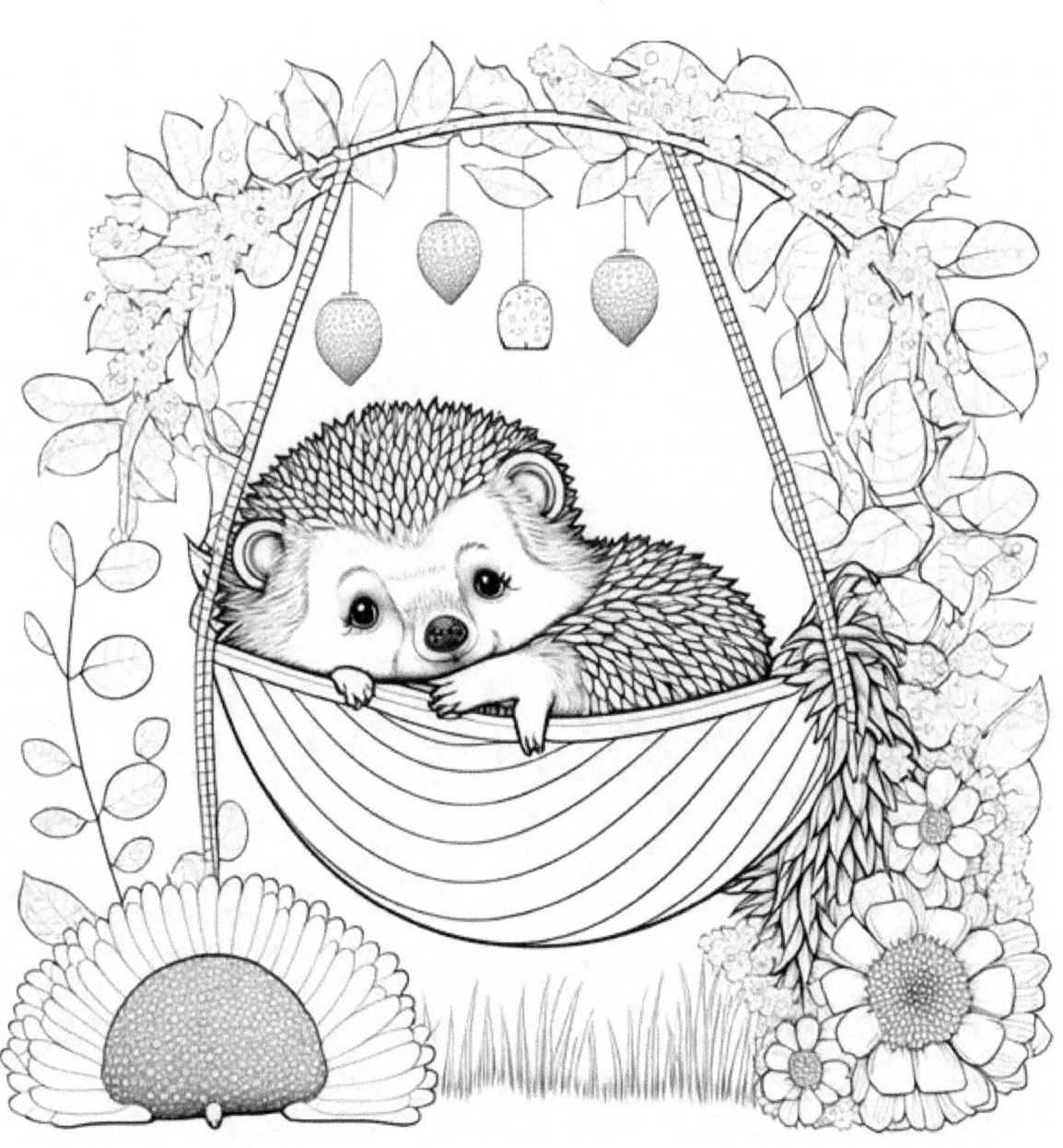

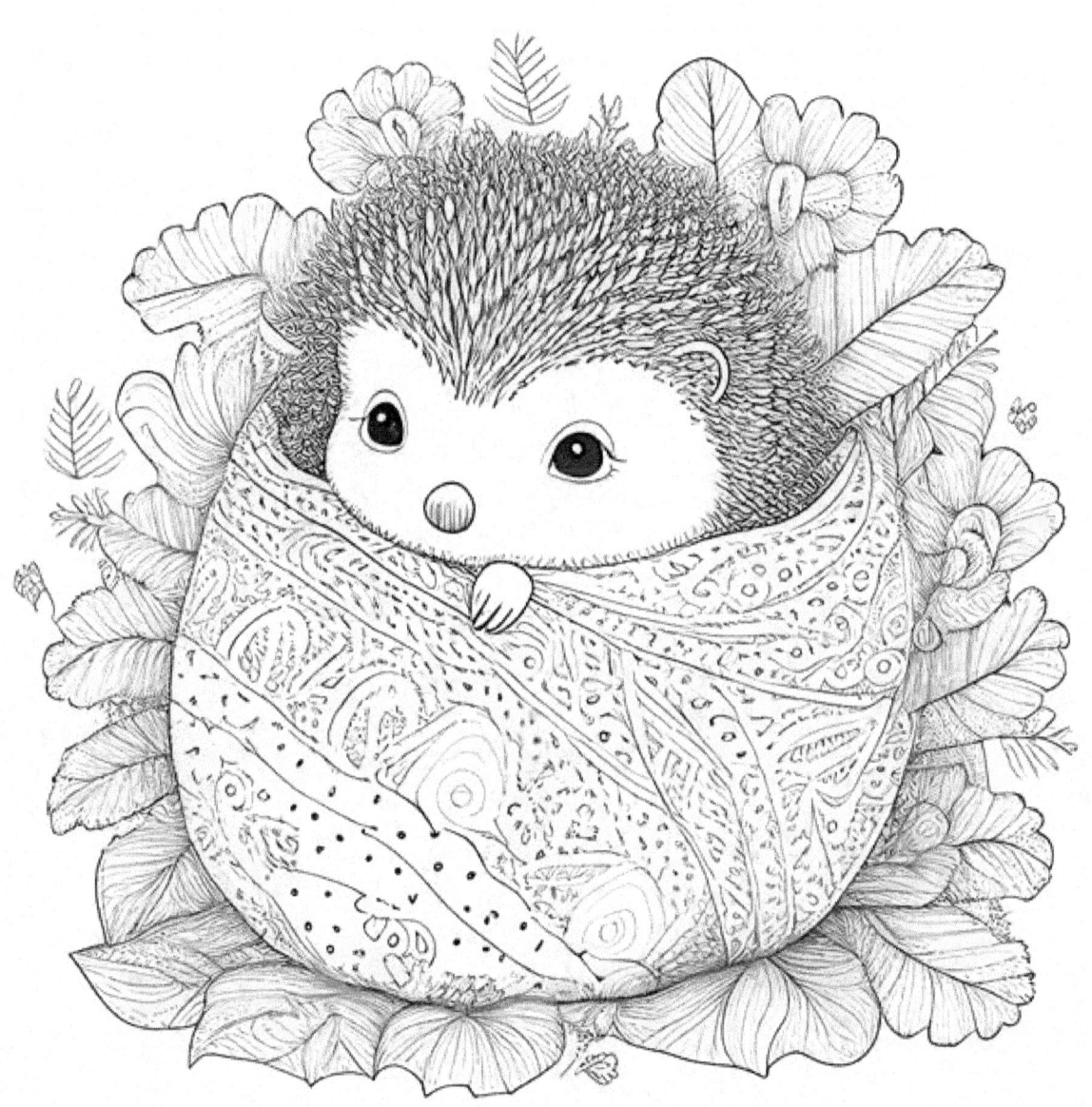

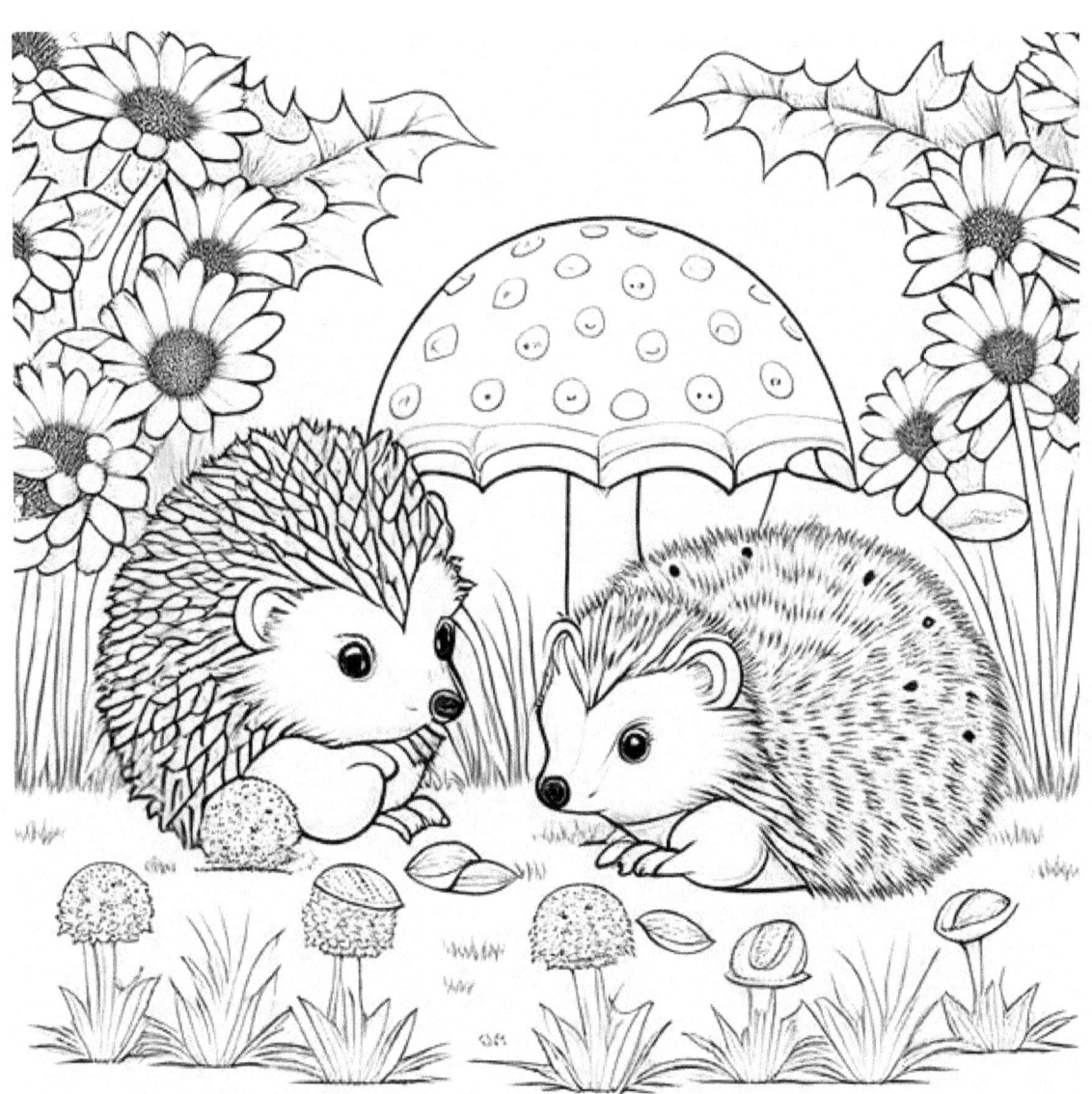

```
J B U D S F O T Z G P A Z Y V
F R E I N O D J B O W P S Q A
R I M I H V S P I N E S X D O
I S A U E E B D A D F S I I V
E T M Y D W S N O U T M X T S
N L M U G Y O Q G I R T E S S
D E A D E W D Q S T Z S T U N
L S L G H P R R O R G T L X S
Y Q X Y O A D L C E E J A R R
S O W F G C P D C F Q D V X L
J N X H E N S T R U N H J C O
U Z Q G M K L N I K T F G C Q
Q R N Y H L F I U V B E L G T
P R R E U Z K Z T G R V T H L
I P R I C K L Y W Z Z X B N G
```

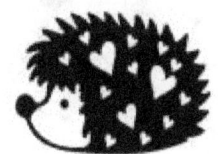

Can you find these
hedgehog words in the
puzzle?

HEDGEHOG
PRICKLY
SPINES
CUTE
MAMMAL
SNUG
BRISTLES
SNOUT
FRIENDLY

Can hedgehogs swim?

Answer: Yes, hedgehogs can swim, but they're not strong swimmers and it's best for them to avoid deep water.

What is a baby hedgehog called?

Answer: A baby hedgehog is called a "hoglet." Mother hedgehogs usually give birth to four or five babies at a time.

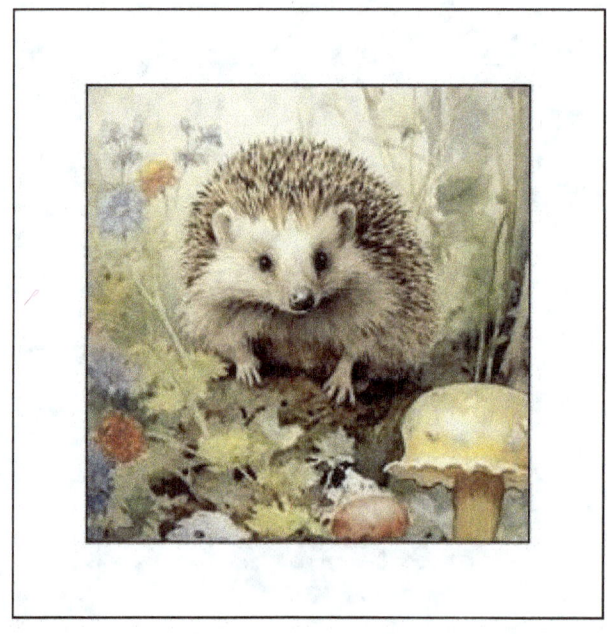

HEDGEHOG JOKES

I shaved a hedgehog once.
It was pointless.

How do hedgehogs kiss?
Very carefully.

What's a hedgehog's
favorite flavor of chips?
Prickled onion.

Where do wizard hedgehogs
go to school?
Hedgehogwarts.

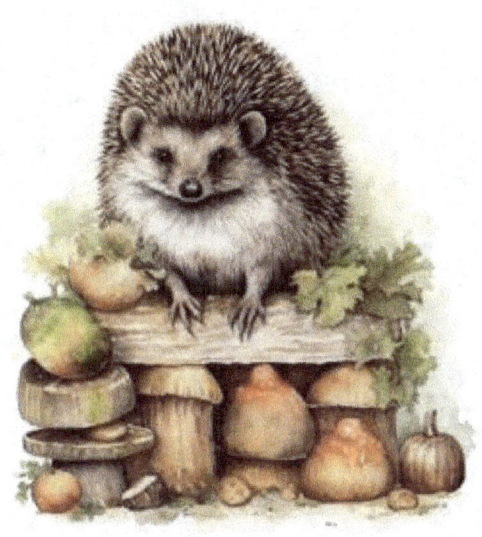

What do you get when you
cross a snake with a
hedgehog?
Barbed wire.

What do you call a
hedgehog that doesn't eat
worms?
A hedgetarian.

Which animal won't share
the shrubbery?
A hedgehog.

Why was the hedgehog told
off in class?
He was being too edgy.

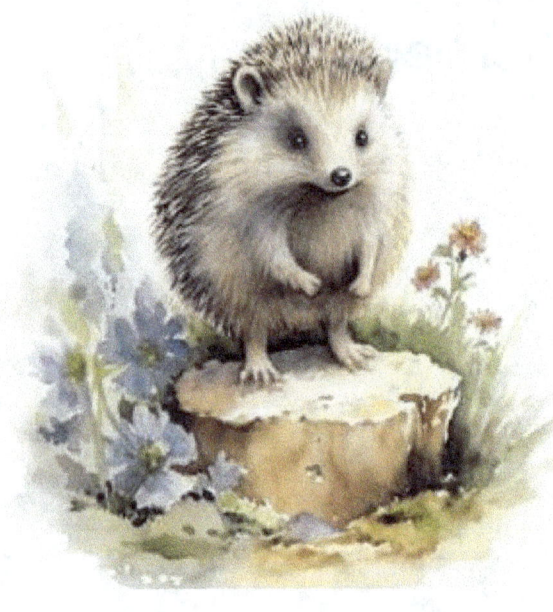

How do hedgehogs play leapfrog?
Very carefully.

What sound do hedgehogs make when they kiss?
Ouch!

What do you get if you cross a hedgehog with a giraffe?
A very long toothbrush.

What do you get when you cross a hedgehog and a pig?
A pork-upine.

What do you call a hedgehog that's lost it's prickles?
A mole.

What did the angry hedgehog say to his enemy?
I will quill you.

What is a prickly pear?
Two hedgehogs.

What do you call someone who buys up the garden store's entire stock of shrubbery?
A hedgehog.

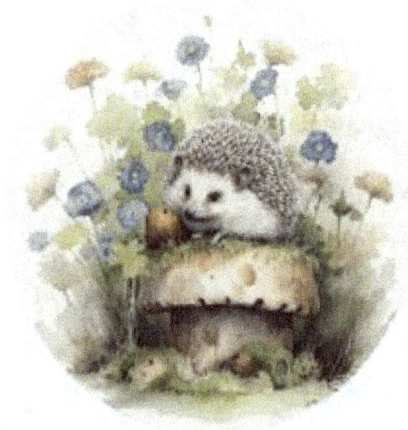

Two toothpicks are hanging out in a forest when all of a sudden they see a hedgehog passing by. One of them shrugs and says,

"Hmm, I didn't even know they had public transport here."

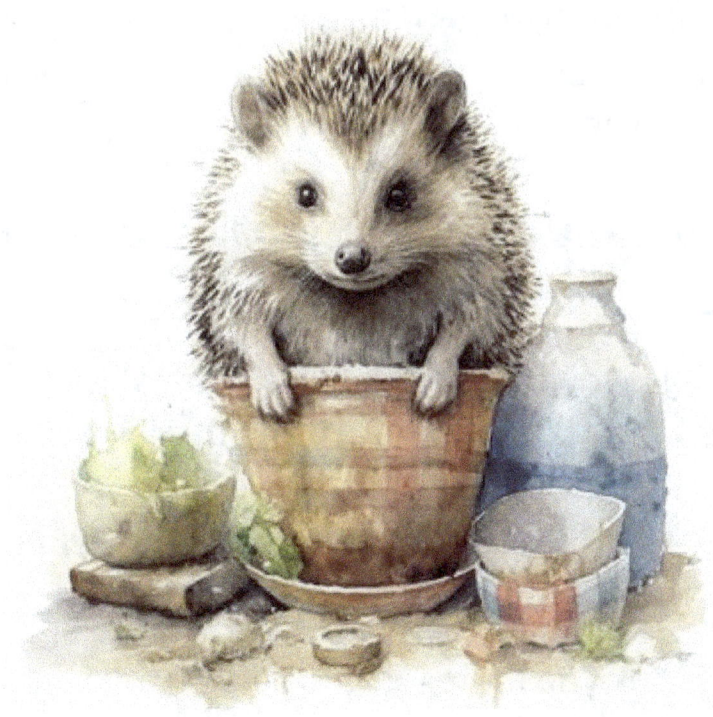

Heather's Hedgehog Hostel
hedgehoghostel@gmail.com
07827751083

Heather's Hedgehog Hostel is a small rescue centre for wildlife, specialising in hedgehog rescue and rehabilitation.

It is a registered charity and is always busy and in need of food donations so her spiny guests can have a healthy, nutritious meal each day.

If you would like to donate food or other much needed items on line you can place an order via their Amazon wish list which can be found here:

https://www.amazon.co.uk/hz/wishlist/ls/28AI0FY2C4W7Q

Alternatively, you can make a one-off donation to help provide life-saving care via their PayPal using this link:

https://www.paypal.com/paypalme/hedgehoghostel

Thank you for reading this book and if you enjoyed it, please consider leaving an honest review on Amazon to help other people learn more about hedgehogs too.